DISEASES OF WOMEN.

DISEASES OF WOMEN:

THEIR

CAUSES, PREVENTION,

AND

RADICAL CURE.

BY

GEO. H. TAYLOR, M. D.

AUTHOR OF "PARALYSIS, AND OTHER AFFECTIONS OF THE NERVES," "EXPOSITION OF THE SWEDISH MOVEMENT IN CURE," ETC.

GEO. MACLEAN,
PHILADELPHIA, NEW YORK AND BOSTON.
1871.

PREFACE.

Many excellent treatises on Pelvic Pathology *and* Therapeutics *are already before the medical profession and the public; yet there are principles involved in these subjects which no previous works discuss or even indicate. I am not aware of any treatise in which the causes even of the ordinary affections of the pelvic contents are distinctly pointed out, nor of any in which the complete cure of these affections is shown to depend on the removal of their causes. I know of no work which maintains the practicability of correcting the faulty position of the pelvic contents by strengthening their natural supports; none in which the possibility of removing pelvic hyperœmia and its consequences by restoring the natural motions of the dominant parts are even referred to, much less demonstrated. This work attempts to supply these deficiencies, and to set forth certain principles which medical literature has overlooked.*

It is a source of sincere gratification that in the development and verification of these principles I have received the kindly support, and often the hearty co-operation, of the profession. The workings and results of these principles prove them to be not merely accessory to, but an integral part of, medical science; a knowledge of them, therefore, becomes a permanent extension, as well as simplification, of the physician's resources, insuring more successful and beneficent results in practice.

Women are everywhere suffering from want of acquaintance with the physical laws of their being. No age or station is exempt. The need of the services of the physician is, to a large extent, due to inattention to and ignorance of principles easily understood and practiced. To point out these principles, and to show how simple, natural and eminently practical they are, has been my purpose. I therefore commend this treatise to WOMEN, *confident of thereby rendering them a genuine service of permanent value. Let no one be discouraged by medical terms, as a Glossary at the end gives their meaning.*

G. H. T.

No. 69 West 38th Street,
New York, 1871.

CONTENTS.

I.

NEGLECTED FACTS IN UTERINE PATHOLOGY, AND THEIR THERAPEUTIC IMPORTANCE.

Mechanism as well as chemistry involved in the vital functions—Mechanical facts afford a distinct order of therapeutic resources.—Pages 13–21.

II.

THE PELVIC CONTENTS HAVE NO EXCEPTIONAL TENDENCY TO DISEASE.

Uterine disease easily prevented, and easily removed—Uterus and appendages less liable than other organs to disease—Unreasonableness of some usually assigned causes.—Pages 22–29.

III.

INITIAL AND DERIVATIVE FORMS OF PELVIC DISEASE.

Liability of confounding symptoms with disease—Pelvic disease passes through progressive stages and successive forms, all depending on the same causes—The various symptoms should not be regarded as different diseases—

The different views of physicians are fragmentary rather than antagonistic—The causes of pelvic hyperæmia, the primary element in pelvic disease—Evidences drawn from anatomy, from physiology, and from therapeutics.—Pages 30–43.

IV.

SUMMARY VIEW OF THE LEADING FORMS OF DISEASE OF THE PELVIC CONTENTS.

Morbid conditions—Congestion, Inflammation, Leucorrhœa, Ulceration, Hypertrophy, Ovarian affection—Pelvic Cellulitis—Morbid Positions—Prolapsus or depression—Inclination—Anteversion—Retroversion—Morbid Functions—Menorrhagia, Dysmenorrhœa, Irregularity—Disease of Ovaries—Subacute inflammation.—Pages 44–56.

V.

CAUSES OF PELVIC HYPERÆMIA, AND OF DISSEASES PROCEEDING THEREFROM.

Circulation of the blood retarded by mechanical obstruction—Effects of perpendicular and horizontal positions—Brown-Sequard—Effects of respiratory and other reciprocating motions on the circulation in the pelvis—The diaphragm a piston, and the effect of its motion on the contents of the pelvis—Effects of twisting motions—Illustration of upward motion caused by twisting—Lifting effect of voluntary actions—What protects the pelvis against accidents—An important point in diagnosis.—Pages 57–75.

VI.

INFLUENCE OF ORDINARY EXERCISES ON THE HEALTH OF THE PELVIC CONTENTS.

What kind of exercises are prejudicial and what are not—

Necessity for prescribed exercises for invalids.—Pages 76-89.

VII.

THE PELVIS AS RELATED TO DRESS.

The motions of respiration extend from the diaphragm downward as well as upward—Effect of obstructing this motion—How dress affects the pelvic contents—Abdominal respiration necessary for health—Dress and civilization—Rationale of female clothing.—Pages 90-104.

VIII.

INSTRUMENTAL SUPPORT OF THE UTERUS.

Supports repress muscular action—Natural support supplied only from above—Objections to the pessary.—Pages 105-117.

IX.

LOCAL APPLICATIONS IN UTERINE DISEASE.

Local remedies do not affect the causes, therefore insufficient and inappropriate—Caustics less effective than other agencies—Various injurious effects of local applications—Opinions of leading Gynecologists.—Pages 118-144.

X.

FURTHER STATEMENTS OF PRINCIPLES AVAILABLE IN PELVIC THERAPEUTICS.

The system an apparatus for generating and manifesting force—The purpose of all medical treatment is to control and increase this manifestation—Force transferable from one region of the system to another, for therapeutic purposes—External force can aid and control the internal manifestation—Active and passive motions or movements. Pages 145-156.

XI.

MEANS OF SECURING SUSTENTATION OF THE PELVIC CONTENTS.—EXAMPLES OF MOVEMENTS.

1. Movement for increasing the space in the superior portion of the cavity of the trunk—2. Similar process for the same purpose—3. Movement for raising the abdominal and pelvic contents, through action of the chest, by apparatus—4. Movement for cultivating the power of the chest, and increasing its control of the parts beneath.—Pages 157–168.

XII.

METHODS OF EMPLOYING GRAVITATION AS AN AID IN RESTORING THE POSITION OF THE PELVIC CONTENTS.

5. Movement for raising the contents of the pelvis, involving aid from gravitation—6. Movement requiring the coöperation of muscular action with gravitation—7. Similar process for the same purpose, but requiring an assistant—8. Movement combining gravitation with muscular power—9. Movement employing the full effect of gravitation—10. Movement employing both muscular action and gravitation, facilitated and graduated by apparatus.—Pages 169–183.

XIII.

MEANS FOR INCREASING THE POWER AND ACTION OF THE MUSCLES OF THE ABDOMEN.

11. Movement requiring action of the abdominal walls at each side—12. The same, aided by an assistant—13. Movement calling into action all the anterior muscles of the abdomen—14. Movement developing the oblique and trans-

verse muscles of the abdomen—15. The same, without assistance—16. Twisting movement of the trunk—17. Movement for elevating the contents of the abdomen and pelvis, and to strengthen the sustaining parts—18. Movement combining the action of the chest and diaphragm, with twisting the trunk.—Pages 184–200.

XIV.

KNEADING THE ABDOMEN.—COMBINATION OF KNEADING, WITH MUSCULAR ACTION AND GRAVITATION.

19. Kneading the abdomen without apparatus—20. Apparatus for kneading, to be worked by other than muscular power—21. Kneading with rollers.—Pages 201–222.

XV.

DEMONSTRATION OF THE EFFECTS OF PROCESSES. PROLAPSUS OF THE BOWEL IN ADULTS AND IN CHILDREN.

Elevation of the contents of the female pelvis—General weakness and pelvic laxity.—*Cases.*—Pages 223–238.

XVI.

CHRONIC MENORRHAGIA.—Cases.—Pages 239–253.

XVII.

HYPERTROPHY AND RETROFLEXION.—Cases.—Pages 254–267.

XVIII.

SECONDARY EFFECTS OF MEDICAL APPLICATIONS TO THE UTERUS.

Uterine complications with spinal disease, its rationale and remedy, illustrated by cases.—Pages 268–278.

XIX.

THE CONNECTION OF NERVOUS WITH PELVIC DISEASE.

Morbid sensation, its causes, varied phases and remedy, illustrated by reference to cases.—Pages 279–293.

XX.

MORBID EMOTION.—HYSTERIA.

Morbid intellection.—*Cases.* Origin and Predisposing causes of Nervous Derangements in females.—Pages 294–316.

DISEASES OF WOMEN.

I.

NEGLECTED FACTS IN UTERINE PATHOLOGY, AND THEIR THERAPEUTIC IMPORTANCE.

A CONVICTION of the inadequacy of the current methods of treating diseases incident to the contents of the female pelvis, and of the importance of recognizing certain cardinal facts and principles which are now usually overlooked both by patients and practitioners, has led to the writing of the following pages.

The chief source of erroneous judgment in this matter is the limited number of known or generally admitted facts. The well-attested facts bearing on the subject are of the utmost importance, but are altogether insufficient to establish sound scientific conclusions. To obtain more facts relating to the subject is therefore a matter of special importance in Etiology, since our ideas of this subject practically control our Therapeutics.

Each of the current medical opinions, of which there is a vast variety, undoubtedly contains a grain of truth. These opinions originated in the different appearances the same thing presented from different points of view; each of them represents some but not all of the facts involved in the subject under consideration. It is therefore reasonable to suppose that the more we increase the points of observation, the more important facts shall we elicit, and the nearer shall we approximate absolute truth. Each new observation, whether it discovers new facts or brings into new relief those hitherto unappreciated, affords a broader and surer basis of therapeutic advantage. In this way real and permanent medical progress is made; while otherwise medical science and practice must remain stationary—tempting targets for whoever wishes to assail them.

I propose to call attention to the subject of Uterine Pathology and Therapeutics from a hitherto neglected point of view, and thus to introduce the reader to facts that are not generally mentioned in works on these topics. I desire to call attention especially to the *mechanical relations* of the pelvic organs, and also to the part these relations play both in the pathology and the therapeutics of the pelvic region.

The existence of such relations has received a passing recognition by the Profession, in some of the means employed in Pelvic Therapeutics. But, so far as I am aware, it has failed to apprehend, much less has it set forth, the true pathological and therapeutic significance of the facts involved in these relations.

The importance of a careful investigation of this field of inquiry is obvious. Were the *mechanical* elements eliminated from Physiology, there would be very little left that would call for discussion. The great functions of Respiration, Circulation, Motion, Nutrition, and the Evolution of Force, both sensorial and dynamic,—*all* involve the idea of a change in place of the matter of which the system is composed. Any adequate consideration of these functions includes a variety of facts pertaining to mechanism, both as regards the form and structure of the vital apparatus, and the force which it exhibits.

In fact, vitality implies mechanism. Even if

we reduce our idea of life to its lowest possible terms, by restricting it to the simplest mode, we shall still find that vital existence is inseparable from mechanical function and activity. The action of this mechanical force has hitherto been held of little or no account; but the existence and influence of this force I propose to make clear. The interplay of chemical force with vitality will, by analogy, aid us in understanding what this mechanical force is and how it operates. When vitality ceases in death, chemistry has entire control over the elements thus abandoned, and in proportion to the decline of vitality in the system chemical force asserts its sway. Medicine consists very largely of materials designed to prevent or to counteract the disastrous effects of chemical force within the living body.

So also the force of gravitation is ever present in the system, and ever asserts its power in proportion as vitality declines in any part of the body. While the influence of chemistry is exercised over atoms, the power of gravitation is exerted over masses. The part gravitation plays in inducing disease, and the assistance it can be made to yield in the restoration of health, form a highly interesting and hitherto neglected subject of inquiry.

It is plain, therefore, that the mechanical relations of the pelvis, and the various forces that are active for good or ill in these relations, should receive thorough investigation. This is specially important in order that pathological causes may be better understood, and that suitable therapeutic and hygienic conclusions may be derived therefrom. If we neglect this field of inquiry, and the important facts that it may yield, it is obvious that our practical inferences, our conceptions of pathology, and our remedial resources will be alike incomplete.

Such mechanical facts, and the principles involved in them, naturally suggest a new order of remedial resources. These differ greatly from the medical appliances in common use, and this may possibly lead some minds to question their value or to condemn them outright. But improved remedies for painful and often fatal diseases can afford to wait for recognition, certainly as long as those who need them. When it shall be found that these remedies are more direct, more appropriate, of more rapid and permanent effect, and useful alike in all the multifarious forms of pelvic disorder—resembling in this respect the air and food which are necessary alike for all—both patients and the profession will undoubtedly cordially welcome and adopt them.

Therapeutic measures for which such a basis and such a wide range of application are claimed, will naturally provoke and should certainly receive the severest questioning. This is heartily invited. Let the facts and principles set forth in these chapters be subjected to the severest tests. I am chiefly anxious to know and state the truth on the subject for the benefit of those who may and those who do suffer. The rejection of erroneous opinions is oftentimes indispensable to the reception of the truth, and so nothing but benefit can come from careful inquiry and the publication of its well-attested results.

Another important advantage should flow from the enlargement of the number of admitted facts bearing on this subject. We shall arrive at a clearer understanding of the relative value of the remedies to which we have heretofore been restricted, and about which there is much disagreement in the medical world. We shall also ascertain the *limitations* as well as the uses of the various remedies. Thus we shall be enabled to avoid their *misapplication*, their *useless* application, and their *abuse*, from each of which patients now suffer much.

Nor need we be deterred from this undertaking by the recent labors and achievements of modern Gynecologists. For though uterine pathology and therapeutics have been elevated to the dignity of a distinct branch of medical science, this science can hardly be supposed as yet to have passed through its progressive and to have arrived at its perfected stage. Indeed, the practical advantages yet derived from the cultivation of this specialty are far less than will be found attainable when the facts involved shall have been turned to proper account. Our knowledge of actual and differential local pathology has been greatly improved; while the *causes* upon which these states directly depend have been most unaccountably ignored. Our therapeutics have hence been directed, *not* to the removal of the causes, but to the palliation of effects. The common results of practice are consequently transient; the actual disease continues while the symptoms fluctuate. While intent on the multitudinous *aspects* of disease we fail to comprehend its essential nature as related to ultimate causes.

The truth of these statements is substantiated by such considerations as follow. The number of females who require the services of the physician in affections of the pelvic contents increases rather than diminishes, as is evident from the increase of specialists devoted to this branch of practice, the supply being proportioned to the demand. The length of time required for treatment, often extending through months and even years, is a convincing evidence of its insufficiency. The persistence of annoying symptoms, after ordinary remedial treatment has been discontinued, and the frequent reappearance of old symptoms after they were supposed to be permanently subdued, are conclusive proofs of the same fact. The frequent change of physicians, and resort to new and sometimes questionable remedies, indicate that neither the cause nor the effects of disease are satisfactorily reached. The fearful increase among females of a great variety of nervous disorders, especially those of an emotional nature, popularly as well as professionally connected with the organs under consideration, strongly intimates that the nervous system endures continuous though indefinable suffering from causes dependent on the condition of this important centre of nervous sympathies.

In the light of the above statements, an important fact is clearly apparent. If it be a function of the physician to develop and diffuse a knowledge of the *causes* of diseases of this class, the failure to fulfill this duty is signal and complete. In some future time such a service may be regarded, as it certainly is, the highest and most important of his calling. Preventive knowledge and preventive measures are here of much more consequence than in the instances of infectious diseases, in which the law provides salutary regulations, because the cases are more numerous, and the aggregate of suffering greater.

The development, popularization, and diffusion of facts bearing on this subject must inevitably result in the diminution of these affections, if not in their entire prevention, as serious and prolonged diseases. It is to these comprehensive and unquestionably important ends that my efforts in the present work are directed.

II.

THE PELVIC CONTENTS HAVE NO EXCEPTIONAL TENDENCY TO DISEASE.

It seems to be the prevailing impression that the contents of the female pelvis are peculiarly liable to disease; in short, that a tendency to disease inheres in these parts, and is liable to development at any unexpected moment. The causes of such disease being constitutional or hereditary, the victims of it are therefore quite free from all responsibility in the matter. And there are physicians who appear to countenance this impression; at least, they do not protest against it, and their silence is construed into testimony in its favor.

This idea must be vigorously combatted and effectually repressed before any real advance can be made in uterine therapeutics. In order to render the sufferer anything more than the most superficial and temporary benefit, *her active co-operation is absolutely essential.* Certainly no one will be likely to contend effectually against a malady which is regarded as in any degree inevitable.

But that diseases of the contents of the pelvis are not inevitable is evident from the fact that the brute creation enjoys entire immunity from them. Brutes are subject to various other diseases, which often prove fatal; but there is no instance on record of any but the human female suffering from diseases of this class. This remarkable fact indicates that the cause of the disease in the latter case is not constitutional, and that women are not necessarily its victims. But it indicates that women should use the knowledge they have abundant capacity and opportunity for acquiring in such a manner as to prevent these diseases and exempt themselves from the sufferings to which they are peculiarly liable. If the animal has an advantage in position, woman has a greater in reason, which is a more powerful protector and guide than any brute organ or instinct of which we now have knowledge. It is only necessary for her to use reason for her own protection and well-being, to enjoy a complete immunity from these painful diseases, which sometimes lead to fatal results.

The position of the generative intestine in women, being chiefly underneath the mass of digestive organs, has sometimes been regarded as peculiarly unfavorable to health. There are considerations, however, that entirely remove this idea, and which indicate that, on the contrary, the location of the pelvic contents is peculiarly favorable to health, showing, moreover, that the purpose of nature to preserve the species, even, if necessary, at the expense of the individual, is well displayed in the disposition of these organs. Such considerations as the following appear to justify this statement:

The pelvic organs are enclosed in a bony encasement, stronger and more capable of resistance than any other portion of the body, consequently these organs are better protected than the brain, the spinal cord, or the chest, and are less liable to injury from accidental and external causes than any other part of the system.

The pelvic contents are also less liable to suffer from causes connected with digestion than most other parts of the system. Placed quite outside the digestive tract, these organs can never be directly affected by irregularities in that process, like the stomach and bowels. The relation of the pelvic to the digestive organs is more remote than that of the muscles and nerves, since they need constant support for the discharge of their functions. Even acute attacks of the digestive organs are seldom communicated to the generative intestine.

The perturbations of climate and temperature sometimes occasion, if they do not excite, various diseases; but they hardly have any considerable influence on the pelvic organs.

The overtasking of the voluntary powers are sometimes thought to affect the pelvic contents unfavorably. A closer analysis of cases, however, has generally shown that this cause, when it has appeared to operate unfavorably, acts indirectly, and through deficiency of nervous and muscular power, the nerves and muscles being the first sufferers from over-exertion. It is quite another class of women than the *workers* who suffer most from pelvic affections. The reason for this important but indisputable fact will hereafter be made plain. The numerous secondary affections arising in acute diseases, it is now well known, fall upon every other portion of the body more than upon the one we are considering.

We have left, as the *cause* of disease of these

organs, the abuse of their own functions. But these abuses affect the nervous system rather than the pelvic organs themselves, and are treated accordingly. The exceptions constitute a separate class of special diseases, which the present work does not propose to consider, and which are outside of the scope of the Gynecologists. Those aberrations of functions, deformities and diseases of the uterus and its appendages for which physicians are daily consulted by the most conscientious and moral women in the community, both married and single, are not regarded by patients or physicians as attributable to abuse of the sexual functions, and are not prescribed for as having such origin. Harlots, and women subject to ungoverned and immoral excesses, are said to be nearly exempt from diseases of this class.

It has been asserted by some authors, that the periodical function of women, which is absent in the lower order of animals, produces a strong tendency to disease of the generative organs. It is thought by some persons that this monthly afflux constitutes congestion, which, under frequently recurring and unforeseen circumstances, merges into disease. A little reflection will show the untenableness of this presumption. This function is as natural as the action of the brain or the muscles. All organs, during their activity, receive alike a large accession of blood. This is a necessary concomitant of any functional act. But brain and muscles do not, as the consequence of their functional activity, have a necessary tendency to disease. Health, and not disease, is the consequence. Disease can only result from a prolonged and excessive activity which constitutes abuse, and generally when from other causes the organs are unfitted for work.

Nature, however, kindly provides against any possible predisposition to disease of these organs from this source in an exceptional manner, as is shown in the method of disposing of the blood of functional activity. In case of every other function, this fluid passes freely on its natural course; in case of this function it is at once excluded from the system. This fact would appear to provide against the probability of disease arising from the cause assigned.

From these considerations it is evident that other causes than those already referred to must be sought for the diseases from which women suffer so frequently and so much. These causes must be co-extensive with the suffering, which is greater and more widely diffused than is generally supposed; and as these causes are probably unsuspected, they cannot be avoided. The apathy of women, even those who suffer most, to the causes of the diseases which produce the suffering is inexplicable; and their willingness to resign themselves to the care of physicians for affections more easily avoided than contracted, and their unwillingness to study the legitimate means and methods of directing those delicate processes of their systems, which they, of all others, ought best to understand, are certainly unreasonable and astonishing.

But suffering tends to work out favorable results in legitimate succession. The first impulse of the sufferer is to seek relief. This is the stage of blind credulity. The victim willingly subjects herself to such other suffering or sacrifice as those in whom she reposes confidence prescribe. If her efforts to obtain relief in one direction fail, she seeks it elsewhere, losing strength and faith with each successive trial. After repeated failures she begins to inquire, "Wherefore? Is this apparent tendency to pelvic disorder real and unavoidable? Can the causes of this prostrating disease be discovered and eradicated? Has not human nature intelligence enough to learn the natural history of this derangement, and sufficient force of will to prevent, if not to cure it? In short, is not this a case where a knowledge of cause and effect is attainable, and where the effect is removable by eradicating its cause?" Such questions intelligent females are beginning to ask with a seriousness and urgency that indicate a determination to have them intelligently answered.

It is lamentable that the public is content with such low aims in matters relating to health. Even many physicians are content to afford their patients immediate but questionable comfort, without sufficiently studying ultimate effects. The natural consequence is that causes are suffered to remain unabated, while effects are experimented upon and the system is tampered with. The disease should be fully explained to the invalid, so that she can comprehend its origin and workings; for without her intelligent co-operation the successful treatment of her case is almost impossible.

III.

INITIAL AND DERIVATIVE FORMS OF PELVIC DISEASE.

CHRONIC diseases of the pelvic viscera differ from other chronic diseases chiefly in location.

We should divest ourselves of any notion of intrinsic peculiarities arising from other sources. All disease, wherever located, when reduced to its last analysis, is the consequence of imperfect vital action. There is some impediment, known or unknown, to the complete expression of the vital power; and imperfectly vitalized products, or non-vitalized material, invade the system, and exhibit their presence and their effects by local disorder.

The great obstacle to the correct understanding of disease, and consequently the chief impediment to its removal, is the too exclusive attention paid to particular modes of its expression. There is insufficient breadth of observation and of generalization. It is too often forgotten that the *manifestation* of disease, whatever it may be, can never exist unsupported; that there is necessarily something back of it, often unrecognized because unsought, but generally detected when earnestly looked for. The symptoms are merely the utterances of this something, which we should seek to ascertain and remove. We commit grave mistakes in considering the symptoms as *the disease*, and restricting remedial attention to them.

Another consideration should be here presented. Disease in general, and that of the pelvis in particular, is progressive in its character, not only in its degrees, but also in its forms. It not only passes through various stages of development, but is liable to become developed in different directions from the same apparent beginning. The different characters thus assumed do not necessarily require a corresponding difference in remedial treatment, provided this treatment be in the initial stage. The commencing stage is necessary to the very existence of disease.

Modern Gynecology has devised the means for thorough investigation of the pelvis, and has made great advances in the determination of actual and differential diseased states. Treatment is, theoretically, applied with reference to the facts thus elicited. But these facilities in arriving at facts have not by any means produced unanimity of opinion among Gynecologists, either in regard to essential facts or necessary treatment. This is because different physicians look for, and therefore find, different conditions. This statement does not imply that anything is really unrecognized by the competent physician, but that superior consequence is attached to special points of pathology, which therefore secure exclusive therapeutic attention.

For example, leucorrhœa, having its seat in inflammation of the glands of the uterus and its connections, is thought by some physicians to be the principal cause of uterine maladies, and they direct treatment for the suppression of this symptom. With others, displacement is regarded as the general cause of all uterine affections, however varying the symptoms. Supporters are, with these, the indispensable remedy. Ovarian inflammation is regarded by other physicians as competent to account for most of the symptoms referred by the patient to the pelvis.

Others still, following Dr. Bennett, insist that it is inflammation of the neck of the uterus which accounts for the symptoms observed; the remedies are consequently exclusively addressed to this easily accessible part. I confess myself to have been an early and faithful follower of Bennett; but the gradual development of the facts and principles presented herein convinced me of the incompleteness and insufficiency of that author's views regarding both pathology and practice. Chronic Metritis is by many looked upon as a more reasonable explanation of both the rational and the physical evidences of pelvic disease than is inflammation of any special tissue or part of the organ.

There is still a respectable minority of physicians who continue to regard all pelvic symptoms, whether physical or rational, as so many evidences of deteriorated general health, and therefore prescribe remedies chiefly with reference to this fact.

Much stress has of late been laid on minute points of pathology, as therapeutic aids, by leading Gynecologists. To designate these differences in the location of points of greatest apparent deviation from health, we find employed such terms as these: cellulitis, endometritis, parametritis, perimetritis, trachealitis, endotrachealitis, &c. The knowledge of these distinctions is evidence of the searching nature of modern inquiry, and illustrates the perfection attained in our means of diagnosis. Their influence must, however, be confined to narrow limits, or they prove damaging to our practice. The too close observance of these special and minute distinctions has these effects:

To circumscribe the physician's inquiries to a local point;

To limit the remedial means to such as may be locally applied;

To ignore the existence of causes upon which the declared manifestation directly depends;

To presume that the effects of topical remedies are confined to the point of application.

This latter is a dangerous error, and cannot but produce untold mischief. It is strange that, in these days of the free use of the hypodermic syringe, through which to produce effects on the general system, this error should have been overlooked.

The differing views entertained by well-informed physicians regarding the chief seat of the difficulty in pelvic affections are not so conflicting and inharmonious as would at first appear. They are detached, fragmentary, and incomplete, rather than antagonistic. They represent different aspects and consequences of the same thing—

various outcroppings of the same subterranean strata. Trace these points of prominence a single step backward, and remove the technical rubbish, and we disclose the same solid foundation. The superficially differing pathological states are then found to have a common origin and starting-point.

The non-professional reader of medical works will be struck with a glaring deficiency in the accounts of uterine affections; very little, often nothing, is said regarding their origin. Writers appear content to describe conditions and remedies; they do not fully explain why and how these conditions arise. They refer to over-exercise, to mounting stairs, to menstruation, to the matrimonial state, and various others as exciting causes. These, however, are but intermediate and secondary. This is apparent from the fact that the great mass of females are constantly exposed to all these and other causes, without detriment. This implies the presence of some other condition; or rather, that the real cause lies in some other fact, which those referred to are capable of rendering operative. We are the more confident that this latter is the correct statement from the consideration that the conditions above mentioned are not in themselves unwholesome, but quite the contrary.

The study of disease will doubtless be more satisfactory if its beginnings be regarded with more scrutiny, and its initial processes be more thoroughly understood. It is not enough that we become familiar with its accumulated effects. We need to watch the point of departure from the full expression of vitality, in order to seize upon its causative influences.

The operations of life constitute in the organism a circuit of mutually dependent processes. We may profitably commence their examination at any point of this circuit, but the most natural and convenient one is the point where inanimate matter becomes living substance, the instrument of bodily force. Here we find the necessary conditions to be the presence of suitable material brought by the capillary blood-vessels. Vital parts are always in immediate relations with these vessels; the materials vitality employs are thus brought—those it rejects are thus disposed of. It hence follows that these vessels have intimate connection with the occurrence of disease, and are immediately responsible for vital conditions.

The paramount use of this connection is the conveying of material; in other words, the *motion* of the fluids bearing the incipient vital substance. The minute instruments of force which, aggregated, form muscle and nerve are organized from material thus derived. These organized structures express their functional power, that is, yield their force, through the agency of oxygen, which arrives through the same channels to the point of use.

We must bear in mind that disease and imperfect and perverted nutrition mean much the same thing. They indicate stages of the same process. The initial stage must be connected with the transformation of non-organized matter to its organic forms. The capillary blood-vessels furnish the conditions whereby these changes are effected. These vessels, therefore, bear most intimate relations to vitality, whose diseased expression may have two opposite forms—*Anœmia* and *Hyperœmia.*

The first of these terms indicates that nutritive supply is insufficient for local needs; it becomes so through deficiency of material, or through deficiency of the causes which carry forward the blood. The deficiency of power and function which characterize anæmia, can hardly be regarded as a local disease, but a general one. The local region would not suffer if the causes derived from the system at large were in complete order. The local symptoms hence betray negative characteristics.

The indications of treatment are very evident. This should consist in increasing the nutritive capacity and action of the system at large. The introduction of more oxygen by respiration requires more food; the blood is enriched. The pelvic region, under these influences, recovers its functional tone, as soon at least as the general system. The condition of the menstrual function may be regarded as affording, in general, very reliable indications of the existence and degree of anæmia.

The superior value of exercises to correct pathological states derived from this source is attested by all classes of physicians. The only question which has arisen is regarding the means of rendering this agent available.

In *hyperœmia*, there is turgescence, or local fullness of vessels, but deficient motion of their contents. The sluggish motion allows some portion of their contents to assume other changes than those of health. Materials obey in part the laws of chemistry, instead of being fully controlled by those of vitality. The wasting matters, those which have served vital uses, are imperfectly elaborated; their contact with oxygen is too feeble; the resulting product—carbonic acid, water and urea—is diminished; intermediate and insoluble compounds appear; there is, consequently, partial retention of devitalized substance. This explains some of the phenomena of uterine diseases; the increase in size, the hypersecretion, &c., of portions of these organs when in a diseased state.

Hyperæmia may be regarded as the chief condition we have to deal with in restoring the health of the pelvic contents. Various evidences of this statement will hereafter appear. For the present it will be sufficient to adduce facts from the following sources, both as substantiating this statement, and as preliminary to the comprehension of the principles forming the basis of the present treatise.

1. *Anatomy.* The pelvic organs are provided with an extraordinary supply of blood-vessels. "Rouget has particularly investigated this subject in a memoir of great value. The utero-ovarian

artery, which supplies the uterus with blood, passes upward. Its first branches, to the cervix, are small; but opposite the body of the uterus it gives off suddenly twelve to eighteen short trunks, which pursue at once a spiral direction and divide into a large number of smaller branches. When injected, these branches are seen to be so close as to quite cover the sides of the uterus. The body of the uterus thus receives a very profuse arterial supply, and the spiral convolutions may be seen projecting into the sinuses of the uterine structure. The veins in which these arteries terminate are still more numerous and capacious, and they form a plexus, covering the body and sides of the uterus."* The ovaries are supplied with blood in the same manner and quite as profusely.

2. *Physiology.* "The purpose of all this capacity for blood is to supply the conditions necessary for procreation. One of the first of these is the *menstrual function.* In the human female, the engorgement and full distention of these vessels occur periodically, the period of engorgement being that of menstruation. Mens-

* Graílly Hewett, on Diseases of Women.

struation is an indication of the fact that the ovaries are in activity; in other words, that ova are being formed, developed and matured in the ovaries. By menstruation is meant the periodical discharge of sanguineous fluid from the uterus; this discharge being attended, as before remarked, with a congested and engorged state of the uterus, ovaries, and adjacent organs; in most cases, by hyperæsthesia of the parts in question."* In health, it is well known, this condition is but temporary. The afflux abates in four or five days, and the vessels of the parts return to their normal condition. In disease, however, these vessels fail to contract sufficiently; they retain an abnormal amount of blood.

3. *Therapeutics.* The most cursory inspection of the works of authors on uterine therapeutics, of the various schools of practice, and through all the progressive stages of development of uterine pathology, indicates agreement in one particular. They unite in proposing remedial measures to relieve the pelvic organs of this oversupply of blood. The means which are recommended to secure this effect may differ very greatly,

* Grailly Hewett, M. D.

while the principle of therapeutic action remains nearly the same. Some may contend for local depletion, some for peripheral revulsion, others may insist on the sufficiency of local or general alteratives of specific virtues; but all agree in the necessity for diminishing the calibre of the pelvic vessels, and relieving their hyperæmic condition. This is regarded as the essential preliminary to the assumption by vitality of the full control of the affected region and its various constituent parts.

4. *Improved Methods.* The peculiar efficacy of the therapeutic methods herein introduced to notice is in good part due to their superior power in the direction above indicated. They afford very great, indeed, well nigh perfect, control of the various causes of the hyperæmic condition. They also cause interstitial mechanical activity. This results in correcting and perfecting the quality of the fluids, and also causes direct and rapid absorption of surplus fluids at any congested point. As these effects produce progressive amelioration of all symptoms, and prove rapidly curative, it follows that they supply still further evidence that local hyperæmia constitutes the beginnings of ordinary pelvic disease.

The fact of the existence of pelvic hyperæmia as preliminary to pelvic disease, is still further substantiated by all evidence indicating an adequate cause. The causes of such a state need not be inferred simply by this effect; they are in no degree hypothetical, but are definite, tangible realities. They are, primarily, *debility, and the consequent deficient action of certain muscles of the chest and abdomen, through which the rythmical motions of respiration are communicated to the viscera;* secondarily, *the deficient support of the weighty and mobile parts superimposed upon the pelvis.*

IV.

SUMMARY VIEW OF LEADING FORMS OF DISEASE OF THE PELVIC CONTENTS.

For convenience, we may speak of affections of the womb and its appendages as consisting of *Condition*, of *Position*, and of *Function.* It must be understood, however, that these terms are not intended to denote several distinct diseases, but the different ways that disease may be exhibited in the same individual and in the same parts. These forms of disease sometimes appear in equal degree, but more frequently one or another preponderates so as to attract special attention and afford a name to the affection.

MORBID CONDITIONS.

Hyperœmia, Congestion.—These terms imply distention of the capillary vessels of any portion of the generative apparatus, whether belonging to the lining or the covering membranes or the muscular or areolar tissues of which these organs are composed. Congestion simply means retention of the circulating fluids in undue amount by the minutest vessels. It implies a diminished vitality, as shown by their imperfect contraction. They are unable to act effectively against the column of blood they contain. While the facility of the progress of the blood *to* these vessels remains unimpaired, or is but slightly diminished, its facility of progress *through* as well as *from* them is more or less impaired by causes yet to be explained.

The ovaries, uterus, vagina, and their lining and covering membranes, or any portion of either of these organs, may suffer from congestion. The various degrees and combinations of this condition in these several parts will, of course, afford a multiplicity of symptoms, according as the sensory nerves are affected or as function is modified. The volitions and the muscular power become implicated in their mysterious connections with the pelvic region according as the congestion merges into other pathological forms. Congestion is preliminary to, as well as coincident with, all pelvic disease.

Chronic Inflammation.—When congestion is extreme in degree or long continued, several important modifications appear, designated by the term inflammation. Some portion of the contents of the distended capillaries escapes through their thinned walls into the surrounding parts, thus adding to the substance of such parts and causing swelling. The occluded circulation also confines the heat produced, thus elevating the temperature; while the fact of these changes is indicated to the consciousness by *pain.*

The distinction between congestion and inflammation is not, perhaps, precisely definable; hence these terms are often used interchangeably, to designate the same condition. The difference is, however, generally regarded as one of *degree* of development of the morbid action, both implying the same initial stages of fullness and over-fullness of vessels. Precision in the determination of these distinctions is not quite possible, nor is it practically called for. The important point to understand is, that the true remedial measures must be such as shall aid the circulation of the fluids of the minutest vessels through the obstructed point.

Leucorrhœa.—When the thinned and weakened walls of the capillaries which permit the transudation of their fluid contents as above described are those of the *lining membranes*, it is readily seen that the fluids thus escaping cannot be retained by the tissues, but must be conducted off. The canal of the uterine neck and the vagina thus forms a channel for such fluids, which, perhaps modified by commixture and decomposition, constitutes the leucorrhœal discharges so common in these cases. The effect of such discharges is to drain off fluids, and thus to relieve the surcharged vessels of the affected region. It is at once the effect of, and relief for, congestion. This is the best circumstance that could occur under these conditions.

The ordinary method of remedying congestion and inflammation of the parts referred to is to *produce* a leucorrhœal discharge, by means of some local stimulant or irritant, applied to the membrane as near as possible to the point where the congestion is most severe.

Ulceration of the lining membrane of the neck and also of the mouth of the womb not unfrequently occurs, but is not so frequent or formidable a matter as is often thought. It consists, in general, in the yielding—"solution of continuity" —of the mucous membrane of that particular locality. This may be regarded as purely the effect of conditions existing in subjacent parts. Its existence serves to palliate the over-congestion that otherwise would exist, but is in no sense to be regarded as a cause, or considered in itself as an evil. Ulceration, contrary to popular and even professional opinion, has no disposition to continue beyond the existence of its cause. We shall show, in the proper place, how easily and certainly the removal of this effect of local congestion and inflammation may be accomplished by restoring the normal relations and fructifying the interior forces of the system. Physicians in this case, also, are apt to resort to remedies quite similar to those before described as employed in congestion, and diminish the local hyperæmia by means of an artificial outward drain.

Hypertrophy.—Should the surcharged vessels fail to be relieved of their accumulated fluids by removal in one of the modes described, and should the cause of congestion continue, the plastic elements of the blood are disposed to assume some low form of organization, and thus become an addition to the amount of tissue, or at least of the substance of the affected organ or part. The size and weight of some portion of the womb, or its appendages, are thus increased.

This effect more frequently occurs in a portion only of the organ, as either the anterior or posterior portion of its *neck*, *body* or *fundus;* or even a more limited part of these divisions.

The ovaries are often subject to similar forms of affection, which are denoted by characteristic symptoms. The relief afforded by leucorrhœal discharge tends to preserve the vagina from the results of hyperæmia.

These forms of disease are almost infinitely varied by location. It is very seldom that the whole of the tissue of the organs or the whole of its mucous membrane is affected. Generally, but a limited portion is subject to disease, while the remainder escapes. Each variation of location will afford variety in the symptoms. A congestion or inflammation of the fundus will give rise to different symptoms from the same condition of the neck. The anterior and posterior portions of either the womb or the neck may also be separately affected. The lining membrane of the body or of the neck may be separately congested, or may afford distinct and characteristic secretion. All these different states depend, however, on the same or similar causes.

Chronic Pelvic Cellulitis.—This may be described as congestion or rather chronic inflammation of the pelvic contents outside the uterus. The affection involves the connective tissue of the broad ligaments and other tissues of the pelvis, producing tenderness, and disabling the female from active exercise or prolonged upright position. The acute form is apt to terminate in abscess. This form of pelvic disease is manifestly dependent on the same causes as those affecting the whole or particular parts of the womb.

MORBID POSITIONS.

Like most visceral organs, the uterus is quite mobile, and cannot be regarded as naturally occupying a fixed position. It not only rises high in the abdomen when gravid, but at other times its location is quite dependent on the disposition of superior and surrounding organs. The limited size of the pelvic cavity, and its lateral ligaments, of course restrict its power of change within certain limits.

The same cause, however, that superinduces the abnormal states previously described, serves powerfully to limit the wholesome range of movement of the womb, and to cause malpositions.

These malpositions consist, in general, either in the *depression* of the organ, or "prolapsus;" its *inclination* forward, backward, sidewise, or in any intermediate direction; or its *flexure*, causing the fundus and body only to point in either direction mentioned, while the cervix remains in or near its normal axis. When the womb inclines or is bent forward, it is called *anteversion;* when backward, it is called *retroversion.* Unless these inclinations and flexures are extreme, the symptoms arising are associated with, and are hardly distinguished from, those of the hyperæmia that co-exists. When extreme, however, the body and fundus of the womb will press upon and interfere with some other part, as the bladder, the sacral nerves, or the rectum. This latter condition produces more painful effects than any other malposition, since it seriously interferes with and sometimes prevents the action of the lower bowel, and for obvious reasons is more difficult of removal than other displacements.

The reader will keep in mind that the above-described conditions are merely *effects*, and have a direct and demonstrable relation to legitimate causes, which, in the light of the facts presented, are removable.

MORBID FUNCTION.

Whenever the above-described conditions exist in extreme degree, or for a considerable period of time, they in turn become causes of *morbid function.* The most important manifestations of morbid function are the following:

Menorrhagia.—This occurs in a variety of forms. The immediate cause can only be dilatation of the vessels from which the flow proceeds. This dilatation occurs in consequence of hyperæmia, previously described. The hyperæmia may be referred solely to lack of the motion which should secure the return or venous circulation; caused either by superincumbent weight, obstructing the return flow, or by a flexure at the junction of the body with the neck of the womb, producing a mechanical obstruction restricting the freedom of flow. Either of these causes produces expansion of the uterine cavity, as well as of its lining vessels. In either case the conditions are favorable for too much flow; in the latter there is also *Dysmenorrhœa,* or unnatural pain, attending the function.

Such deviations of function as too great periodical frequency, intervals or periods too prolonged, and irregularities in general of the menstrual act, are of minor importance, and are referable to the same general causes, modified by temporary deviations of health, occasioned by reasons too complex to be estimated, such as temperament, personal habits, occupations, mental and emotional influences, etc. The successful treatment of each of these, as well as other varieties of pelvic disease, should evidently be conducted on the same general principles, but modified to suit individual idiosyncrasies and temporary emergencies. Such treatment will consist in restoring the natural motions of the parts involved, and the effective removal of the superimposed weight.

DISEASE OF THE OVARIES.

On account of the location of the ovaries they admit of less facility in examination; and the beginnings of disease in these organs are more obscure than in the rest of the generative intestine. It may reasonably be inferred, from their simplicity of form and their known physiological action, that such beginnings of disease would be *hyperæmia,* followed by *subacute inflammation.*

Moreover, the rational inference, from certain peculiarities of symptoms in females suffering disease of the pelvic region, is that these organs are affected in the way described, either primarily, or as participating in known affections of the uterus. It is perfectly reasonable to infer that the same and identical cause, operating alike upon both organs, should induce the same form of disease in either or in both, and as nearly alike, in kind, as their structure will allow.

Owing, however, to the lack of mucous secreting surface, their hyperæmia is *not* kept in check by an abundant watery discharge, as in case of organs with cavities. The ovaries are, hence, liable to a form of disease peculiar to their structure, as distinguished from that of the rest of the pelvic contents. This is dropsy. We can hardly conceive of the co-existence of this form of disease with the presence of active venous circulation, leading the blood freely away from the affected parts. The blood readily yields its watery constituents in case of obstruction, or the least impediment to its onward flow. The true way of removing accumulated watery fluids from the ovaries, as from any other part, is to secure *venous absorption.* This is sure to occur whenever the venous circulation is urged forward by means involving no reduction or exhaustion of vital power. The means of accomplishing this result, it is readily seen, are identical with those required to remove the weight of superimposed organs from the pelvis, the principles and methods for doing which are hereafter to be explained.

In the above sketch of affections incident to the female pelvis I have mentioned only the leading forms of such disease, and have not intended to include all the numerous varieties or degrees of severity that are liable to come under a physician's observation. Such detail would not further my purpose. This is confined solely to the development of the facts and elucidation of the principles involved in the special therapeutics herein set forth; while those involved in other therapeutic procedures are intentionally neglected. It is the first principles rather than the details of pathology that are, in this treatment, brought into requisition, and concerning them it is presumed there will be substantial agreement. For it can hardly be conceived but that disease, of whatever form, must have its beginnings in perverted nutrition, having an origin and resulting in consequences something like what I have described. And though disease of the different portions of the pelvic viscera may, and indeed often does, run into various pathological forms by the accumulation of secondary pathological products, yet the true principle of cure must continue to consist in measures which most powerfully antagonize the perversion of vital energies, and lead them in the proper channel. These must always be such as shall vivify the circulation and all the functions therewith connected.

V.

CAUSES OF PELVIC HYPERÆMIA AND OF DISEASES PROCEEDING FROM IT.

THERE is no difficulty in observing and understanding the effect of a ligature applied to an extremity. In the phenomena thus arising we have a good illustration of the conditions existing in various pelvic disorders, and of their causes. The flow of the current in the vessels leading from the extremities to the heart is obstructed by the pressure thus supplied; the retarded blood accumulates before the obstructed point in an amount proportioned to the completeness of the obstruction. The series of consequences which inevitably follows from any similar cause is something like the following:

The arterial or outward flow is but little interfered with by such a cause; hence the venous vessels continue to receive blood in the usual way. The larger vessels soon become filled and distended, and this fullness reacts upon and involves the minutest capillaries. The walls of these latter vessels thus distended become thinned and weakened, lose their contractile power and control over their contents.

In this condition of the capillaries, the tendency of their contents to escape into the surrounding tissues is vastly increased. This tendency exists in health, for interstitial nutrition is carried on by means of the material thus furnished. But in health the amount thus passing the capillary walls is strictly regulated by the demand created by tissue-change. When this escape is not duly regulated, the phenomenon of swelling occurs.

In the imperfect mechanical and vital conditions now described it is apparent that the coincident chemical changes will also be incomplete and imperfect. Both the amount and the degree of chemical action is, under these circumstances, diminished. The chief, ultimate products of chemical action under the control of vitality are carbonic acid and water, most of which escape from the system in a volatile form. Incomplete products do not readily thus escape; hence the *heat* product attending these changes is retained, giving rise to another of the phenomena peculiar to inflammation.

These effects are always accompanied with more or less pain. This consequence of morbid action may be the result of different causes. The pressure exerted upon the sentient nerve by the swelling is probably one cause of pain. The change in temperature may be another. An undoubted cause of pain in chronic cases is the altered nutrition of the nerve substance resulting from the new chemical products arising in the process described; a cause which points distinctly to its proper remedy in the restoration of healthful nutritive action.

Such are the first but inevitable consequences which speedily follow any cause operating to obstruct the sanguineous flow, whether this cause be experimental or morbid. The aggregate of these effects is in proportion to the completeness of the obstruction and the length of time it may continue.

If a similarly obstructed condition should occur in the vessels of a portion of the body which we cannot directly see and handle, as some part of the contents of the cavity of the trunk, we can easily understand that a similar series of morbid phenomena would occur, as the direct and inevitable consequence of such mechanical obstruction. If we *knew* of the existence of the obstruction, the existence of the effects would be patent to our reason. When we are certain of the effects, should we be less confident of the existence and nature of the cause? Given a *hernia* or *phlegmasia dolens*, and our conclusions regarding causes are definite and unalterable. We are not content merely to palliate symptoms, but undertake, as our first business, to remove, as far as we may, the obstruction.

Now the morbid conditions I have described as existing in the pelvis, affecting either all or some portion of its contents, are as similar to the series of effects produced by mehanical obstruction as the structure of the parts will allow. The *effect* of ligature may, of course, be produced by *any* pressure upon circulatory vessels, through *any* agency capable of supplying such pressure.

There are two causes whose direct action, either separately or combined, is capable of delaying the circulation in the pelvic vessels. One of these is hydrostatic pressure—gravitation of the contents of the venous vessels. This in turn is traced to insufficient action of the causes which return the venous blood, allowing it to remain sluggish in its vessels, especially the venous capillaries. The other cause of pelvic hyperæmia, and also of the displacements and deformities that have been described, is the superincumbent weight of overlying abdominal contents, pressing upon the pelvic viscera. The movement of the circulation in these parts is thus mechanically obstructed.

It remains to be shown that the causes named are abundantly capable of producing the effects now ascribed to them; also under what circumstances they operate, and on what conditions they in turn depend.

EFFECTS CAUSED BY POSITION.

Only in the human species does the longitudinal axis of the body correspond with the perpendicular. The human female is *erect*, while all other animals support the trunk parallel with the horizon. In the absence of restraining causes, the effect of position is easily seen. The weighty contents of the abdomen gravitate toward the abdominal walls, or toward the pelvis, according to the position in which the trunk is placed.

The pelvic cavity is continuous with the abdominal, and in the upright position the contents of the abdomen, being exceedingly mobile, readily obey the law of gravitation. The broad *pelvic bones* and the *abdominal walls* furnish support to these contents, *but supply no obstacle at the superior opening of the pelvis to the effect of gravitation upon its contents.* Hence, the necessary effect of this position is to subject the contents of the pelvis, which are located in the inferior portion of this continuous cavity, to the pressure of all the superior organs. The pelvic contents must, therefore, in the absence of muscular action, furnish some degree of support to the overlying parts.

In the *horizontal* position, such as is assumed by animals, this effect of gravitation is essentially reversed. The abdomen is now pendulous from the spine; its axis is horizontal, and actually *lower* than that of the pelvis, though parallel with it.

The tendency of gravitation of the abdomen is consequently to drag the contents of the pelvis forward and downward, *from* the pelvis *to* the abdomen. The effect of this position is not only to remove the weight which otherwise would fall upon the pelvis, and, with the weight, all its effects upon the position of the pelvic organs and circulation in the pelvic viscera, but also to make some degree of traction upon the organs within the pelvic cavity.

The fact of the influence of position on the condition of the pelvis in certain degrees of the bodily weakness here brought to prominence, is amply confirmed by the universal tendency of females thus afflicted to assume the recumbent position. This affords a speedy relief, because it removes at once the vascular hydrostatic effect, and also the superincumbent visceral weight. If the invalid lies with abdomen downward, so that its weight shall *draw from* the pelvis, a still greater degree of relief is experienced.

The above statement regarding the effect of gravitation in the upright position the reader will understand, refers only to the effect of *unantagonized* gravitation. That healthy females have no cognizance of the effects of gravitation here described, is because with such these effects do not exist. The vital mechanism is so contrived that it *as effectually opposes gravitation and its ill effects, as it does ordinary chemical affinities* within the vital domain. So that, in judging of the effects of these causes, we have always to estimate them in their varying relations with vitality.

Gravitation is now referred to as an undeniable power, and as such demanding recognition in pathology. This power is as inevitable in the body as the operations of chemistry. Like chemistry, its effects are good or ill, according as they are directed. Whenever either of these forces is not properly controlled and directed by vitality, as they are not when the vital power has become weakened, it is the function of medical science to afford the needed direction. Chemical faults and deficiencies are legitimately remedied through chemical instrumentalities. Why should we attempt to remedy morbid conditions, arising from gravitation, by irrelevant agencies?

This recognition of the positive influence of gravitation on the contents of the pelvic vessels and on the pelvic organs is not new. Every physician who "sends his patient to bed" on account of pelvic symptoms, aggravated by walking and standing, recognizes this fact, and hopes to abate the effects arising therefrom by the recumbent position. He may never think of using the same power for a curative end that has been productive of mischief, but that power is waiting to do his bidding.

The power of gravitation has been fully utilized in various other medical as well as surgical affections as a remedial agency. Dr. BROWN-SEQUARD * strongly recommends the employment of position as an important element in the treatment of *Chronic Myelitis*, a chronic inflammation of the spinal cord. He says: "Whether at night or in day time, if he lies down, he ought to place himself on the right or left side, and if he can, he should even lie flat on the abdomen, *so as to diminish, by the effect of gravitation*, the amount of blood in the spinal cord. Every physician who has, in this respect, adopted the above suggestion, especially if he has tried it in the absence of other remedies, can testify as to the remedial effect of the position described in the particular class of cases referred to."

Whether the influence of gravitation upon the contents of the pelvis is prejudicial or not depends on other concomitant facts, the chief of which is the vital contractile power of the muscles. The effects of gravitation are completely neutralized when this power is at its height, but as the vital force diminishes, gravitation as well as chemistry gain the ascendency in the system. The restoration of vital contractile power to the muscles of

* See Dr. Brown-Sequard on Paralysis of the Lower Extremities, page 75.

respiration effectually prevents hyperæmia of the pelvic vessels, and consequently all the effects flowing from this condition.

EFFECTS OF RESPIRATORY AND OTHER RECIPROCATING MOTIONS ON THE CIRCULATION IN THE PELVIS.

The actual effect produced by the cause above described depends upon *whether it be continuous or not.* If a ligature applied to an extremity be quickly removed, the temporary obstruction serves to stimulate increased contraction of the walls of the vessels, whereby their contents are more vigorously urged forward. Such an act is, in fact, *exercise,* and serves to invigorate and increase the nutrition of the walls of such vessels, through which their strength and power are maintained.

The vessels of the extremities are habitually changing their hydrostatic relations with every different position assumed by them; sometimes bearing a column of blood, and again relieved of its pressure, according to the varying voluntary actions of the individual. All this is doubtless favorable to the nutrition of the vascular walls, and enables them more perfectly to perform their functions.

But if, by reason of *continued* obstruction in the return circulation from any cause, the blood accumulates in and distends the vessels, hyperæmia is produced,—swelling, heat, pain and effusion, either into the intercapillary substance, or upon a free mucous surface, are the ultimate, inevitable consequences. These effects are, however, normally prevented in women, by the *incessant oscillations* of pressure, caused by the motions of respiration. The consequences of this are similiar to those above described, as arising from change in position of extremities, though probably far greater in degree, as well as more rapid, regular and constant.

If we attentively observe the motions of breathing in any animal at rest, we shall acquire a tolerable idea of the mechanics of respiration. We shall see that the *greatest apparent motion is at that portion of the body nearest the hips.* The body appears to expand and contract at this region, synchronously with every inspiration and expiration, and more than at any other point. It becomes evident that the change of volume caused by the addition and subtraction of a quantity of air in the chest, is propagated through the diaphragm to the abdomen, whose anterior walls participate equally with the diaphragm in this motion.

This action and its effects will be more clearly understood if the diaphragm, which separates the chest from the abdomen, is regarded as a *piston*, having a regular and constant pump-like action. In this way, it draws in and expels air at its superior side (aided by the coöperating muscles of the chest), while at its inferior side it subjects the contents of the abdomen to a similar degree of motion, the volume of the latter remaining uniform.

It is easy to see the effect of this oscillating motion, derived from breathing, upon the abdominal contents. The degree of gravitating force precipitated upon these parts undergoes incessant changes. The abdominal and pelvic cavities being continuous, this effect reaches the pelvic organs, and extends to their minutest capillaries. The action derived from the motions of ordinary healthful respiration maintains the nutrition, contractile power, and tonicity of the capillaries of the whole of the pelvic contents, effectively stimulates the return of their blood to the chest, and secures a due and constant renewal of vital force in these organs, and thus insures their healthful functions.

The influence of this upward motion, caused by respiration, is by no means limited to the contents of the circulatory vessels. The power in question is evidently exerted in equal degree upon the *mass of the pelvic viscera* also. It actually contributes a distinct sustaining power, and aids in maintaining these organs in their normal position against opposing circumstances. The proof of this is complete and practical. It consists in simply augmenting the influence under consideration. Increase the pump-like action of the chest, and it will be found that the displaced pelvic viscera will return to their normal position. This fact evidently affords an important suggestion as to the legitimate means of *cure* for the class of invalids suffering from pelvic disorders, the application of which will follow.

EFFECT OF TWISTING MOTIONS OF THE TRUNK.

We have seen that the upright female, in comparison with the lower animals, suffers a disadvantage in having the abdominal weight *above* instead of *below* the pelvis. The latter, it is plain, can never incur the diseases of the pelvic viscera so easily acquired by the former. Creatures of limited capacities seem to be properly guarded by a beneficent Creator, while increased powers are attended by a corresponding increase of responsibilities.

But, on the other hand, the upright position affords advantages which more than compensate for these acknowledged disadvantages. These arise from the *facility with which the upright trunk may be twisted upon its axis.* A *creature* supported by four legs is utterly incapable of executing this class of motions, while man performs such motions in great variety, with the utmost ease, and with great advantage.

The act of twisting deserves to be carefully studied with reference to its effects upon the contents of the pelvis. These effects may, perhaps, be more easily understood if illustrated by an appropriate mechanical apparatus.

To this end, let us take a piece of inch rubber tubing, six inches long. Provide this with a tight plug at either end, into which insert the ingress and egress pipes of a common elastic syringe, furnished, as usual, with induction and eduction valves. An inflexible axis, whose length corresponds with the distance between the plugged ends, is so placed within the tube as to press hard against the inside of these ends, so as effectually to prevent their approximation under pressure.

Let now one end of the apparatus, thus equipped, be firmly held by one hand, while, with the other hand firmly grasping the other end, a twisting motion is given the tube. The effect of such a twist is to diminish the calibre of the tube and to force its contents out through the eduction valve and pipe. If the induction pipe be connected with a vessel of water, the fluid will be drawn into the pipe and tube, on relaxing the grasp, and will be forced upward in proportion as twisting motion is repeated.

The trunk, mechanically considered, is a similar apparatus. The spine entirely prevents any shortening effect from all twisting motions. The ribs prevent the chest from being contracted by the same acts. It follows that the diminution in size produced by all twisting motions is necessarily confined to the region of the abdomen. Indeed, the chief muscles called into action by such motions are those of the abdomen. The cavity of the chest meanwhile remaining quite expanded, the pressure upon the abdominal contents forces them upward, moving also in the same direction the contents of the pelvis.

The practical inferences, from the preceding explanation of the mechanical functions and uses of the body, may now be intelligibly made.

1. *The abdomen should participate in the ordinary motions of respiration.* Whatever restricts the communication of this motion to the abdominal region is physiologically reprehensible and supplies to the contents of the pelvis a potent cause of disease and deformity; since in this case there is *constant* instead of interrupted pressure, preventing the free return of the venous circulation.

2. *The power and habit of twisting the body upon its axis should be carefully maintained.* If through faulty habits of life such motions are discouraged or neglected, the effect of gravitation in the upright position will not probably, under such circumstances, be fully counteracted. The muscles of the chest, and especially of the abdomen, become weak, flabby and distended, and afford little or no aid in sustaining the contents of the abdomen, and elevating those of the pelvis; and a vastly increased liability to those diseased conditions under consideration becomes the inevitable consequence. The certainty and extent of disease may be regarded as in the

ratio of the *degree of deficiency* in the respiratory and twisting motions.

It may be objected by those to whom the present application of facts is new, that the influence of respiration in the region of the pelvis is too inconsiderable to produce effects so important as are here ascribed to it. But it must be considered that, in fact, the number of respirations, as well as the time of their continuance, is practically unlimited. It is, therefore, not the sudden and transient, but the prolonged and *cumulative*, force that is operative. While the objection stated might hold good as to the effect of a few repetitions of the respiratory act, it completely fails when this act is multiplied without limit, and becomes in effect perpetual.

It may also be objected that the *lifting* effect of the voluntary actions described is quite inadequate to secure so important a purpose as it is here insisted is secured by them.

This objection is refuted by observing and carefully comparing the health of women occupying different spheres of life, or those pursuing the different avocations where twisting motions are, and where they are not, necessitated. Biddy who sweeps and scrubs, and performs many other acts which *twist* her body, enjoys a good degree of immunity from such diseases; placed in the position of seamstress, in which she leads the apparently easy life of constant sitting, she gradually but quite surely loses the power of abdominal respiration, diminishes in size at the waist, and soon enough acquires the forms of disease which affect her distinguished mistress.

It may be well to notice another possible objection to the principle here set forth. If the contents of the pelvis are so affected by superincumbent weight, what protects these parts from serious harm arising from *sudden* disturbance of their momentum, as in accidental falls, in jumping from a carriage, etc.?

The reply to this objection is furnished by the anatomical conformation and relations of the spine, abdomen and pelvis. It will be seen by an examination of the skeleton, that if the line of anterior aspect of the vertebral column be extended, this line will meet the anterior pelvic bones. And, as though it were to render protection the more certain in such cases, the uterus is situated quite under the promontory of the sacro-iliac junction. It therefore follows that any sudden impulse downward must inevitably be guided by, and be in the direction of, the anterior line of the spine, forward as well as downward, so that the shock would be wholly received by the pelvic bones, and *not* by their contents. The operation of such a cause would hence only excite a powerful reactive stimulation, from which benefit would be more likely to be derived than injury.

It is the slow and insidious causes that mainly influence health. As the constant dropping wears away the rock, so will unobserved faulty habits abridge the power of the muscles and nerves, undermine the general and local health, and lay the foundation of diseases most difficult of cure. The causes of diseases of this class are unobserved and neglected, because they are so minute in their beginnings and so insidious, though certain, in their constitutional and remote effects. It is only by understanding the aggregate power of these causes that we become impressed with the necessity of beginning at their origin to remove them, rather than attempt to neutralize effects, while causes continue in unabated force.

The fact of the co-operation of the abdominal with the chest motions in respiration, can hardly be overmuch insisted on. It holds as true in the human race as in animals. The abdominal walls regularly rise and fall with every respiratory act, showing that this act is propagated through intermediate structures and reaches the pelvis, in whatever position the body is placed. This is easily proved, simply by placing the hand upon the abdomen of a healthy person; it will be observed to rise and fall at each respiratory act.

Upon this fact depends an important principle of diagnosis in pelvic diseases. If a female who is a subject of any of the modifications of the diseased state now under consideration, be submitted to this test, it will always be found that the result is negative—*the abdomen is quite undisturbed by respiration.*

The inference from this is plain and direct, that an important principle of cure, in all cases of this class, is *first to restore these deficient but natural motions.*

The reason for the usual persistency of diseases which affect the female pelvis may now be plainly seen. The remedial measures most usually adopted have a degree of irrelevancy. For however appropriate these measures may be in their immediate relations to the effects of these diseases, they generally leave the causes thereof unnoticed or but imperfectly remedied. Permanent health cannot return till those natural and oscillatory or reciprocating motions which have been described, and which are more or less completely suspended in disease, are restored. The return of these motions does not readily, and may never, occur spontaneously. They require special and direct cultivation. The muscles, especially those of the chest and abdomen, are the instruments of these motions. The means of bringing out the power of these muscles require to be systematically studied and applied, if we hope to reach the desired radical results.

While the causes assigned in the foregoing pages for affections of the contents of the female pelvis have been generally overlooked or neglected, other causes have been regarded as competent to produce the effects described.

Those most commonly assigned are such as these: Parturition; Abortion; Displacements; injuries from Pessaries; sudden Cessation of the Menstrual flow; efforts to prevent Conception and, to produce Abortion, &c.

It is proper that these causes should be briefly noticed and their place and value determined.

The first two of the causes above named are

natural processes; they involve a natural and healthful ending as well as beginning; they therefore do not entail diseases. If the return of equipoise and health does not properly occur, and with due rapidity, this fact is conclusive evidence of previously existing pelvic hyperæmia, and its causes. The turgescence of the pelvic vessels continues, because the conditions for removing this state are not in proper action. It hence follows that the above named are, at most, but secondary causes. As to displacements of every kind, their very existence, together with the fact of the employment of supporters and the effect of supporters, prove the pre-existence of the very facts I have stated as the original cause.

Efforts to prevent conception and to produce abortion consist of the most powerful means that can be devised to superinduce pelvic hyperæmia and its consequences. Those who employ these means understand this fact, for the degree of medical knowledge necessary for such understanding scarcely requires special training. Those who submit to these means should, of course, expect to suffer the legitimate consequences of such acts.

The sudden cessation of the menstrual flow in the non-pregnant woman, like the sudden stoppage of any other habitual evacuation, is conceded to be sufficient cause for local congestion and its consequences. But it remains to be proved that the pelvis is more liable to suffer in this case than any other region, if there were previously existing health in these parts. My own observation indicates that so far from being more, it is really less liable to disease from the cause named than are the head, chest, or spine.

It will hence be seen that the causes so commonly credited with producing uterine and other pelvic diseases, growing out of hyperæmia, are merely secondary, and themselves merely effects of certain causes lying behind them, whose nature is perfectly intelligible, and for whose removal there are legitimate remedies. It is also apparent that remedial treatment addressed to these secondary causes, while it may secure temporary palliation, can have little or no permanent effect, since the real disease-producing cause continues in spite of all such efforts.

VI.

INFLUENCE OF ORDINARY EXERCISES ON THE HEALTH OF THE PELVIC ORGANS.

Motions of the body and of its parts proceed from two principal causes. One of these is the influence exercised by the will over the muscles; the other is spontaneous, proceeding from organic needs, independent of the volitions. Deficiency of the motions originating in both these sources has been referred to as causing pelvic hyperæmia and its effects. It has also been seen that the proper support of the contents of the pelvis is equally dependent on the same motions, and that displacement is a natural and almost inevitable consequence of their absence. These statements imply, at least theoretically, that the restoration of due capillary contractility, and of the needed support, may be secured by the supply of motions adapted to the peculiarities afforded by these cases.

This conclusion apparently contradicts the

experience of women afflicted with this class of affections. Such invalids usually regard exercise as prejudicial, feel that it makes them worse, and believe that if it be not the cause of their maladies, at least it aggravates them.

No statement regarding exercise is worthy of notice until it is reduced to a definite form. Exercise admits of an infinite variety in kind and in degree. The body consists of many parts having different functions and relations with other parts. It follows that the application of exercise would produce an endless variety of effects, depending of course upon the diversity of its modes and of the relations of the parts to which it is applied.

The sentiments so freely expressed by invalid women respecting the prejudicial effects of exercise are evidently the product of deficient discrimination on their part, especially as regards the above-named diversities; they show an entire unconsciousness on their part of the radical differences of form and manner of exercises, and the different localities and organs they affect. The ill effects undoubtedly derived from exercise in some cases, especially in affections of the contents of the pelvis, show how great is the need of the utmost care and discrimination in its use. No other circumstance relating to the health of these parts is of greater consequence.

The idea and practice of exercise by such persons are usually confined to *walking*, or attending to some easily performed and non-muscular act in the upright position. There is in most cases an almost entire absence of exercise, except of a very few muscles. But if the pelvic organs be affected by disease, even though it be only in the initial form, previously described, such action is liable to be followed by prolonged fatigue, and a peculiar persistent pain which is referred to the loins, the limbs, or the pelvis. The inability to exercise, which is the so constant symptom of pelvic affections, refers, then, simply to the absence of all exercise, except the non-muscular. No light whatever is thrown upon the action and effect of the almost infinite variety of forms of exercise not employed, and of which most of these invalids are entirely ignorant. Exercise should not be condemned while but two or three of its myriad forms have been tried.

The cause of the suffering, and of the consequent prejudice, alluded to in this special case is apparent. It arises from the relations assumed by the womb and its appendages to the muscles which raise the leg. Some of these muscles have an interior origin, and their contraction produces mechanical disturbance, and therefore pain in the organs, which are already sensitive from disease. Such action also causes an increased flow of blood to the acting region, and in consequence will increase the hyperæmia previously existing. Consequently the avoidance of exercise is not, at first, caused by deficient muscular power, but by fear of pain which is liable to be induced thereby.

The *consequences* of inactivity are, however, disastrous and far reaching. To be deprived of the expression of power through the muscular system, is to lack the most important condition of health. In opposition to her desire, such a person is compelled to lead a life of physical inactivity and listlessness. The unused muscles shrink in size, in power, and in their nutritive supply, while their connection with the *will* becomes more and more enfeebled, till it finally becomes difficult for one so circumstanced to *think* in the direction of muscular activity. Vital power being cramped and confined in the direction in which it most naturally and easily finds expression, necessarily finds scope through the sensations and emotions. The sensory powers become morbidly active, and physiological vigor degenerates into objectless, nervous excitement. The victim of this condition becomes daily more helpless and hopeless, and drags on a most miserable existence for an indefinite period, feeling compelled to refrain from all exercise, the helpful as well as the injurious.

It is a radical mistake to avoid exercise in general because it is found that certain kinds are, under the circumstances, prejudicial. The consequences above depicted result from ignorance or thoughtlessness as to the proper mode of employing exercise. When this subject is properly understood, it will be seen that the suffering described is less a consequence of exercise taken than of that omitted. Exercise is a power as potent to elevate as to depress, and as effective in directing the vital support *from* as *to* any region of the organism. Ill results come from its use being left to accident or caprice, instead of being governed by intelligence.

The force of these statements becomes apparent whenever they are reduced to practice. Let us subject any act, as that of *walking*, to physiological examination. Power, generated by the vital system at large, is, in this act, expressed through a few muscles in a circumscribed region.

Now, in proportion to the expenditure of vital power, is there an increase of the local conditions for its support, resulting in an afflux of blood, freighted with the necessary proximate principles, to the acting part. The supply of nervous energy is, in a similar ratio, increased, and the organs contained by the pelvis become the chief recipients of these effects. These causes are particularly calculated to arouse the consciousness to any condition of disease that might exist; and if long continued without antagonizing or modifying influences, are even capable of superinducing the hyperæmia from which diseases, as we have shown, chiefly take their beginning.

Let us make sure of the principle now illustrated, and see if we may not turn it to good account. It is probable that the same effects would follow from the same causes throughout the system. If the circulation, nervous force, and nutritive materials are thus easily directed to the pelvis, they may also be directed as easily to other regions,—away *from* as well as *to* the pelvis—and become as complete a therapeutic as a pathological cause. In health, the equal exercise of all parts of the body produces an equilibrium of the different parts. In disease, the unequal exercise of selected parts is needful to attain the same end.

Now, it is susceptible of easy and practical demonstration that those very exercises which are often avoided by women as objectionable, and even regarded as pernicious, may, under suitable and prescribed conditions, become not only innocuous, but agreeable and wholesome. To secure this end, it is only necessary to employ such *other and additional exercises* as shall co-incidentally employ a due proportion of the circulation and nervous influence in other and remote parts of the body. By complying with this condition, the afflux to the pelvic region is reduced to the normal quantity, or, indeed, to any extent desirable. *Nutrition and nervous supply follow absolutely and closely on demand*, whatever direction this may take. The maintenance of health becomes hence a problem of maintaining the equipoise of the physiological system through the *intelligence* and *will.* And it will be found that exercises may be so selected as to comply with a variety of therapeutic indications in chronic diseases. They may be so selected and adjusted to the conditions of the system as to quite obviate fatigue, instead of producing it. Indeed, exercise may be so applied as to remove fatigue when already present.

The kinds of exercise that are competent to produce these special results are such as attract the blood with energy *from* the spinal cord; and such as shall secure the *elevating* and sustaining effects that have heretofore been described as the consequence of the action of certain muscles. When such exercises are dexterously employed, not only will the liability to pelvic disease be obviated, but even a pre-existing condition of hyperæmia, the common origin of all pelvic difficulties, will be relieved. Actual and radical benefit will accrue to the suffering part if *general* exercises, embracing especially those that secure action of the chest and walls of the abdomen, are freely employed. But local hyperæmia and its possible consequences are likely to occur, with all their train of prolonged miseries, if *only* such muscles are habitually used as tend to converge the circulation in the pelvic region, without any compensatory or revulsive effects.

To state the principle more definitely. A female may stand, walk, work the sewing-machine, mount stairs, and perform many other exercises usually proscribed as harmful, not merely with impunity, but with actual benefit, provided she does not neglect the motions of the trunk, chest, and diaphragm, which are called forth by many ordinary household occupations, like sweeping, dusting, bending the trunk in other besides the forward direction, *provided* always that these are duly proportioned to the strength.

Call into service the transverse and oblique muscles of the abdomen, and all the muscles of the chest, and the removal of the superincumbent weight from the pelvic organs, and the unobstructed circulation of the blood are thereby assured; the oxidizing process, so indispensable to the evolution of power and the removal of dead matter, is secured to its full extent, and vigor and health to the full measure of the individual's constitutional capacity are the natural consequences.

The practical difficulty regarding the occurrence of pelvic diseases, also the successful means of cure, hence appear to be reduced to very narrow dimensions, easily comprehended. The exercises usually engaged in by females occupying independent positions in society, are altogether *too restricted in kind, and too monotonous in character*, to serve any considerable purpose in maintaining or restoring health.

For this deficiency there is but one real and sufficient remedy. This is, the employment of certain *prescribed* exercises, adapted to the several varieties of cases most frequently occurring, and easily learned and executed. Recourse to this means will, under ordinary circumstances, not only obviate the evils previously set forth, but often also actually secure restoration in cases where disease has not been too long fixed in the pelvic region, on supposition that the muscular strength has not too far deteriorated.

When the deterioration of power has proceeded so far as to render prevention and self-help out of the question, the case is still hopeful, and often not even difficult. The same principles are involved, requiring only prescribed means, and the helpful aid of others.

VII.

THE PELVIS, AS RELATED TO DRESS.

THE regular reciprocatory motions caused by respiration, of which the diaphragm appears to be the centre, have been shown to extend in both directions from it—*downward* as well as *upward*—thus producing an undulating or wave-like motion through the entire contents of the trunk. This fact is easily confirmed by observing closely the reciprocating motion in healthy men, women, or even animals, as it appears externally.

It has also been insisted that this motion does not relate alone to respiration; that it is equally essential to the performance of the functions of the other organs situated in the cavities of the body. The digestive organs require the gliding action of the different contiguous parts upon each other. This stimulates their muscular nutrition and action, and aids the progress of the digesting matters in their passage along the canal. It also promotes the absorption of digested products by the veins and lacteals.

The influence of this motion in maintaining the health of the contents of the pelvis, has already been explained. These contents require the *alternations* of pressure produced by the pump-like or lifting effect of this motion. This action relieves the pelvic contents of the effects of continuous pressure arising both from the weight of the superior or abdominal organs and of the column of fluids in the circulatory vessels. This kind of motion also obviates any tendency to an impacted condition, which otherwise is liable to occur, and is particularly influential in securing vigor of circulation and nutritive action of the pelvic region.

The failure of the motion now described *is in itself a pathological condition.* It is always diminished, and sometimes quite absent, in disease of the pelvic organs. It will be clear to any one who studies these principles that such failure stands demonstrably in the relation of principal cause to disease of the pelvic contents. Other causes doubtless have their influence, and determine largely the kind of effect produced, but have little influence in comparison with the one now stated.

It becomes, therefore, a matter of gravest interest to investigate all the influences which may promote or hinder the extension of this important motion to the contents of the pelvis; for it is these causes which determine the health or disease of the pelvic organs.

The effect of external resistance to this spontaneous motion is obviously immediate and great. If the hand of one person press upon any part of the chest of another, the attention of the person receiving pressure is strongly directed to that point, affording it a greater degree of nervous stimulation, and the heaving motion of the chest at that point is momentarily increased. If, however, this pressure be continuous, the stimulus referred to gradually dies away, and when quite gone, it will be found that a contrary state exists. The muscles and nerves have become wearied, and the motion of the compressed part is diminished. When continuous resistance is applied to the whole circumference of the diaphragm, the respiratory motions of that portion of the chest are of course abridged, and if the resistance be strong, the motion at that point may be quite extinguished.

A critical observer will notice, however, that

when the lower circumference of the chest is compressed, the motions of its upper portion, as indicated by the movements of the shoulders, are slightly increased. A recent medical writer has suggested the probable healthfulness of tight lacing, since it drives respiration to the apex of the lungs, distending the air-cells of that portion most liable to receive tubercular deposits, thus protecting the lungs from disease. This theory might demand our attention if it were also shown that respiration was actually facilitated and enhanced by this means.

That this effect is clearly impossible may be inferred from the mechanical disadvantage at which respiration is in this case performed. The chest resembles a pair of bellows; the greatest motion is at the greatest distance from the nozzle, near which the moving sides are hinged. It is plain that the strength required of the operator is least when he seizes the handles. If he should attempt the labor at any point nearer the nozzle, the power required would be proportionally increased. Compression about the waist would hence require a vastly increased amount of muscular work to expand the chest, since its upper muscles only are employed, if indeed, it be possible for the effect to be thus produced. Any one, by looking at a skeleton and noticing how closely the ribs are united with the sternum, will see that this mode of working the chest is most difficult, if not impossible. If the capacity for motion existed, the muscular power required could never be adequate to perform respiration in this manner.

The mechanical effect of compression can easily be illustrated by means of a common toy. If a thin rubber capsule, containing air, be pressed between the thumb and finger, it will be seen that the part most distant from the pressure becomes most distended and thinned; if the pressure be increased, a rupture occurs at one or both ends. The effect of pressure at the central portion of the body is manifestly similar. Its greatest effect will consequently be at the inferior end of the cavity—the pelvis. Not only are the natural motions of its contents stopped, but the superior parts are crowded down upon them, producing the effect of a ligature upon their circulation.

The indirect effect of deficient respiration on the pelvic organs, which is another of the consequences of pressure, should also be considered. This effect, extending throughout the system, is shown in diminished nutrition of the muscular system, in venosity of the blood, and consequent aptitude to congestion at any weak point, in imperfect digestion and deteriorated general health. All these conditions react on the important and sensitive centre of life we are considering.

There is abundant reason for believing that the *repressive influence of faulty dress* is responsible for much mischief to the pelvic organs in the manner above stated. Garments too tightly fitting, and arranged for continuous and uniform pressure, can hardly fail to aggravate the diseased condition when already existing, and, joined with other circumstances or alone, are peculiarly favorable for the production of all those diseases affecting the contents of the pelvis. It must be confessed, however, that it is difficult to isolate and establish the effect of this cause in a particular instance. The influence of dress is one whose effect constantly changes, not only with the variations of the external cause, but also with varying internal conditions and the general strength. One may stagger under a burden at one time which might be easily borne at another. The estimate of the influence in question must, therefore, be wholly made from a rational point of view.

The opinions of the invalid, with reference to the effect of attire, are quite unreliable; and were we to credit her statements, we should believe that the make and fit of garments, in any individual case, have no influence whatever. In response to our inquiries she affirms *her* dress to be *very loose*, and not in the least to impede the motions of respiration. A triumphant exhibit of sufficient space between the outer and inner garment to insert the hand confirms these affirmations, and impertinent medical cavillers are compelled to silence.

Women, and especially girls, are self-deceived, rather than deceiving, in this matter of the fit of garments. Such demonstrations of breathing space as above referred to are generally unconsciously made during the *expiratory interval*, and the expiration may, unwittingly, be slightly exaggerated, the more certainly to win the point. If required to show the respiratory space at the *inspiratory* interval, the result would be more instructive, but less gratifying, to such as really desire to fulfill physiological requirements in this respect.

Women should bear in mind that it is not the absolute size of the chest, but *the extent of its motion*, that determines the degree of healthful effect produced on the pelvic contents. It is the *fixedness* of the walls of the chest that is deprecated. The communication of motion to the lowermost portion of the trunk always requires cultivation, in order duly to maintain, as well as to restore, the health of the pelvic viscera.

We have a right to call in question the qualifications of women suffering any form of pelvic disease for judging of the physiological propriety of garments. The motions of respiration in this class are but feebly, if at all, communicated to the inferior portion of the trunk, and even the compression of tight garments can but little impede the motions which scarcely exist.

There is a show of truth in the asseveration of such persons that tightly fitting garments do not impede *their* respiration. This, however, is not because their garments are so large, but because their respiratory power is so small. Respiration can never become natural and wholesome while it has such an impediment as a tightly fitting dress to overcome. Even after its removal much time and special attention are required to restore this function to its normal and healthy condition and afford immunity from pelvic troubles.

The reader is warned that attention given solely to the respiratory muscles of the chest will be of little use. It is the co-operative abdominal muscles that are principally at fault, and that require equal, if not superior, attention. It is easily shown that voluntary efforts to deepen natural respiration by such subjects become speedily wearisome, and are soon abandoned. The motion must be involuntary to produce the desired beneficial results. The *will*-power is insufficient to overcome the impediments to brisk respiration for more than a few moments, and the abdominal walls resume their usual motionless condition after such special efforts.

Physiology teaches that so important a function as respiratory motion is not entrusted to the possible caprices of the volitions. These motions need to be performed as well when we sleep as when we wake, and under all circumstances. Even the variations required of this function are under another control than that of the will. When more oxygen than usual is demanded, as under exposure, or increased muscular activity, respiration involuntarily becomes more profound, in exact proportion to the natural or artificial needs, without our knowledge or even notice.

It hence appears that the application of these principles to improve the health of the abdominal and pelvic region cannot be made through any *direct* interference of the attention and will. Direct efforts to expand the chest and elevate the diaphragm are exhausting and useless. The object is secured only by systematic cultivation of the muscles upon which these duties devolve. It must first be ascertained that there are no exterior impediments, and then the abdominal and thoracic muscles can be subjected to all the various motions of which they are capable, both passively and actively, always having regard to their effect on the nervous system.

In proportion as these muscles become hard and strong is the innervation also regulated and strengthened, and each part naturally assumes its proper duties. Respiration takes the abdominal form, and the liability to hyperæmia of the pelvic contents, and its grave derivative consequence, is dispelled, digestion is invigorated, the return circulation is aided, the arterial flow assisted, congestion removed, the contents of the pelvis mechanically sustained, and the health of these parts assured beyond peradventure.

It is plain that in proportion as the habits of females are sedentary will be the disadvantages arising from compression caused by garments. It is on this class that the insidious effect of repression more particularly falls, and they need to be warned of the source of the injury which they so fully experience but so little suspect. A serious degree of compression is quite incompatible with active habits. Modern civilization is popularly regarded as having ameliorated the condition of woman. She is not the kind of slave she once was. But it hardly proves to be of advantage to her, in matters relating to her apparel. It is evident that civilization has much to achieve for her in this respect. The dress of woman has gained little, but has lost much, in regard to comfort and health, and the service it renders her in attaining the objects of life. The customs of civilization compare rather unfavorably with those of less advanced people in this particular. These poor results are attained, not because there is too little thought, said, and done respecting female apparel, but because much of this force is expended in a wrong direction. These faults of female dress are adverted to, because they are directly involved in our general subject. In fact, faulty dress is probably more of an impediment to the physician in the special department of which I am now treating than in all others.

These obstacles to health may be summarized as follows:

The weight of the dress falls chiefly upon the hips and abdomen, instead of being equally distributed over the whole body. It consequently supplies *continuous* pressure (while the woman is in the upright position) against the walls of the abdomen, the part which has least ability to bear it, and where such pressure is productive of most injury. The constant pressure serves to discourage and ultimately quite repress the respiratory motion which should be communicated to the abdominal walls, and thus to superinduce the consequences in the pelvis previously described. The *voluntary* muscular motion of the abdominal walls incident to ordinary occupations are repressed equally with the *involuntary.*

In collecting the greatest amount of clothing about the lower portion of the trunk, (which the style of modern civilized dress demands,) the conditions for maintaining the greatest heat of those parts are also supplied. The effect of such an unequal distribution of bodily temperature is, if possible, more prejudicial to health than is that of unequal weight. The heated parts are necessarily the *relaxed* parts, the parts unstimulated by wholesome alternations of temperature, and consequently the parts in which vital operations are least brisk and vivid. The muscles become the softest and weakest of any in the whole system. But the effect is by no means confined to the muscles. The walls of the vessels are relaxed in equal degree, lose their contractile power, and become unable to resist any tendency to congestion that may come from other causes, but rather favor all such tendencies.

Another objection to ordinary female dress, of quite as much importance as the preceding, arises from its form. It involves a disadvantage of which the wearer of male attire can have but little conception. I refer to the continued imprisonment of the overburdened and overheated parts. There is none of the facility for quick fastening and unfastening that affords so much comfort in the male attire; no contrivances for momentarily graduating its pressure, or otherwise relieving its monotony without resorting to a complete change. If there could be *oscillation* of temperature at will, or at the dictation of the feelings, much of the harm arising from dress would be obviated. Change of temperature of the skin, when not extreme or unwholesomely prolonged, serves to stimulate respiration, quicken dormant vital action, increase nutrition, and affords a wholesome tonic to circulatory vessels.

Many of the disadvantages arising from the present standard methods of female dress might easily be obviated by simply introducing facilities for graduating the fit, so as to correspond with the frequently varying needs arising from daily changes of the weather, and perhaps still more from changes arising within the body, derived from its varying activity, the state of the digestion, and the infinite amount of interplay between these agencies and causes.

Another part of ladies' dress prejudicial to health should be noticed. This is the prevailing style of high heels for shoes. The effect of unnaturally raising the heels and stretching the insteps is to bend the knees forward and hips backward, necessitating a compensating inclination of the trunk. This position not only injures the bodily symmetry, but presses the abdomen down upon the contents of the pelvis, causing the usual train of consequences. High heels also compel the ankles and toes to sustain the bodily weight in an unnatural position, and often prove injurious to the joints.

From the nature of the case the wearer of a garment is the one responsible for the effects it may produce, because she is the only one who can really know much about its fit. Whether she immolates herself on the altar of society and its customs depends on herself alone. The physiological principles involved are easily understood, and are too plain and direct to be easily mistaken. The physician can only represent the consequences, but unfortunately his opportunity to do so does not often occur until the worst has been accomplished that mistaken notions and bad examples can inspire.

VIII.

INSTRUMENTAL SUPPORT OF THE UTERUS.

Malposition of the uterus is a frequent, indeed, an almost constant, element of uterine affections. When the deviation from the correct position is considerable, it becomes the chief object of medical regard, and has stimulated the devising of various forms of apparatus designed as remedies.

These mechanical contrivances are designed to sustain the uterus from below. They usually consist of variously constructed props, or scaffoldings, on which the uterus can rest. Some of these forms of apparatus are quite elaborate and complicated; they are adapted to internal as well as external use, and some combine both.

The *external* appliances are usually so adjusted as to afford upward and inward pressure at the hypogastrium, immediately over the pelvis. To secure this, bands of fabric, rubber, steel, or a combination of these, are passed around the body, and arranged so as to obtain counter-pressure either from the back or the whole surface thus encompassed.

This upward and inward pressure upon the abdominal contents produces, at first, a very comfortable feeling, which is well calculated to deceive in regard to the ultimate consequences. The abdominal contents are held up, and the sense of dragging is relieved, while the removal of weight previously sustained by the respiratory muscles seems to improve respiration.

But if the effects of external instrumental support are still further examined, it will be found that the motion of the contents of the abdomen derived from respiration is effectually prevented. The necessity for action of the muscles which afford this motion has been superseded. While the abdominal contents are securely held up by *external* mechanism, the *vital* mechanism is allowed to drop into disuse.

The reverse of this I hold to be the correct method of reasoning and of practice. It is the vital support that should be jealously maintained, to the exclusion, in the main, of any method of repressing and discouraging vital action. The use of the instrument most decidedly produces the latter effect.

The respiratory and the supporting muscles, being thus relieved of all incitement to action, gradually become weak; and the victim of this treatment very soon finds herself utterly dependent on this false support to enable her to move about the house, or even to endure the upright position. A patient of mine had worn supporting instruments for nineteen years. She was aware of the injury it had inflicted upon her, but was utterly unable to disuse it, so attenuated and paralyzed had the supporting muscles become. Another patient, deceived by the apparent support afforded by an instrument, caused the bands to be tightened till the supporting pad over the pelvis was quite imbedded in the soft structures of those parts. She was obliged to keep in bed, except when the instrument was buckled tightly.

An examination revealed, what it must in nearly all cases of this kind, that the body of the uterus was crowded down and kept down by the pressure of the instrument quite below the position it would otherwise occupy. This organ was pressed so strongly upon the bladder and rectum as seriously to interfere with the function of micturition, and to render natural defecation quite impossible. In this case, whatever there was of disease pertaining to this region was certainly aggravated and perpetuated by this form of treatment; and so deceived was the victim in regard to the cause of these effects that it was with the utmost difficulty that she could be prevailed upon to abandon the use of her instrument.

These cases are not at all unique ; every physician of much practice meets with similar ones. Many are doubtless perplexed for the means of affording health instead of providing such miserable, temporary, and ineffectual make-shifts as supporters prove to be.

These statements do not exaggerate the influence and the ultimate effect of external instrumental support, Such support deprives the uterus of its natural support, and, instead of restoring, it tends to and actually does displace the organ. It not only prevents the nutrition and diminishes the power of the abdominal and respiratory supporting muscles, the *real* support, but prevents the natural oscillating motion of the contents of the abdomen and pelvis, which we have shown to be essential for maintaining the circulation and preventing congestion of these parts. Even the minutest capillaries suffer from diminution of the contractile power of the muscular elements of the region so repressed, and hyperæmia is the inevitable consequence. With hyperæmia, and the effects of gravitation aggravated rather than restrained by the instrument, serious disease of some portion of the pelvic contents—the rectum, bladder, or uterus—follows as an easy and natural result.

The other mode referred to, of affording instrumental sustentation to the uterus, is by means of the *pessary.* This instrument is designed for introduction into the vagina; it finds lodgment at its circumference in the soft surrounding tissues covering the pelvic bones. The form of pessary most in use is that in which the neck of the uterus is allowed to drop through the opening of the instrument, by which means the axis of inclination of the organ is in some degree corrected.

It is evident, from the anatomical conformation of these parts, that no support whatever is afforded unless the mechanical adjustments are such that the instrument is sustained by the pelvic bones. In a large number of cases in which I have removed the instrument (usually superfluous in my treatment) this mechanical adaptation did not exist, and the instrument was consequently of no use whatever, and often lies loose in the vagina. Even if there be most perfect adjustment, it is impossible from the nature of the case to maintain the uterus by this means at only a certain and very moderate elevation—in fact, considerably less than actually exists when the health is restored, and the legitimate sustaining powers rendered capable of doing their work.

An instrument of this sort may with propriety be temporarily used in certain rare cases; such, for instance, as when it may aid in correcting extreme deviation of the axis of the womb. But even in these cases it should be regarded as a temporary recourse, not as a primary or curative procedure. The employment of the instrument is based on an inadequate conception of the condition for which its aid is invoked; not till the laws of the economy are reversed can complete results flow from inferior aims. The fact heretofore shown must be recognized, that the primary disease consists in weakness of those parts upon which the uterus and its appendages depend; and that the local affection in these cases is secondary and derivative. It therefore follows that disease is not so much *cured* as *concealed,* when the treatment consists chiefly of instrumental support.

That invalids of this class are so commonly allowed to use the pessary argues the limited resources at the physician's command rather than his confidence in its curative effect. Its use fulfils at least his desire to do something, or to *appear* to do something, in response to his patient's continued entreaties for help.

But in employing this form of support, the physician apparently ignores the fact that he acts counter to obvious natural principles. He should recognize these facts,—that the pelvis more resembles a tube, with its inferior extremity open, than an enclosed space; that, in reality, the inferior boundary of the pelvis is the one that nature practically leaves open; that whatever support is required in the healthy woman comes from the opposite direction; and that the most effectual support that is possibly available, to any useful extent, consists simply in bringing into healthful relations and active use the *muscular* support with which every living woman is already provided.

But the pessary, as commonly used, is not merely supererogatory. In numerous cases which I have seen, and which, doubtless, exist in every community, it is a positive and effectual hindrance to restoration. The modes in which it acts deleteriously may be enumerated as follows:

1. If of sufficient dimensions to answer its intended purpose, the pessary maintains an extreme distention of the vaginal walls. It entirely prevents, and in time destroys, the contractile power of these walls. The non-contractile pessary is but a sorry substitute for this loss of function.

2. The constant presence of a foreign body in the vagina, actually exerting pressure, not only upon its walls, but the surrounding tissues, is a profound cause of irritation of the whole pelvic region. This pressure exerted upon vessels hinders the flow of their contents, and causes distention of their remotest twigs; exerted upon muscles, it prevents their action, and they become shrunken and useless; exerted upon the mucous membrane, it causes irritation and an abundant and debilitating secretion of mucus and even of purulent matter. This latter determines a corresponding flow of blood to the membrane from which so much is lost; consequently a larger supply is conveyed to the pelvis than is compatible with its health, producing a tendency

to congestion of some portion or all of the region, involving ultimately all the progressive stages of pelvic disease.

3. The hypersecretion described does not consist merely of fluids ; it implies a proliferation of cell-growth on the secreting surfaces—a vital act; and doubtless carries with it a loss of much vital power, which would otherwise be available for functional uses.

4. The products of secretion into the vagina, being composed of mucus, albumen, and an abundance of cell-walls and saline matter, are viscid, and tend to adhere to the foreign body with which they come in contact. Thus they are quite beyond the reach or influence of the ciliary action, which, under ordinary circumstances, duly drives superfluous secretions forward to the vaginal outlet. These matters, therefore, necessarily suffer decomposition within the vagina. The products of this decomposition are liable to absorption, thus adding systemic disease to the local. They react on the vaginal membrane, cause irritation, and are often the cause of a "solution of continuity," or ulceration of any portion of the mucous membrane, which, from other causes, may be rendered liable to this consequence.

5. The pessary is liable to change the malposition of the womb into one more difficult to remedy. While this instrument does not relieve the pressure upon the pelvic organs coming from above, it supplies an additional pressure from the contrary direction. The womb actually becomes "doubled up" under these two opposing forces. Permanent incurvation of this organ is not the unfrequent consequence, which, in the form of retroflexion, becomes a far more serious affection than the original difficulty.

6. Not the least of the evil effects of the pessary is that visited upon the nervous system. The complication of nervous with uterine disease will receive attention in another place; but it is proper here to say that this condition, existing to an extent most difficult to be remedied in ordinary cases, is greatly aggravated by use of the pessary. Its presence is, rationally, an unfailing stimulant to the sensory function of the pelvic region, which powerfully reacts upon the general system. There is no doubt, too, that the absorption of the toxic principles generated in contact with the vaginal walls may be as influential in increasing and perverting the sensations as a similar cause would be at the digestive surface.

The attention becomes directed and finally morbidly fixed at the local point and source of pain, and the whole mental power becomes narrowed in proportion as it is drawn into this exclusive channel.

But the local pain is more than paralleled by the havoc made with the general nervous system. The indefinable uneasiness, the backaches, headaches, the nervous startings and shudderings, the depression of spirits, and the hysteria that make up the life of a woman so afflicted, would render it a terror to be a woman if all this were as necessary and inevitable as it appears to be.

Uterine supports have been devised in which the supporting part is held in place by its connection through a stem with an external band. This form of instrument is mentioned here because it presents the specious recommendation of obviating some of the ill effects above enumerated, viz., pressure upon soft parts, upon vessels and bones, and over-distention of vagina.

These objections are, however, only remedied in a degree, and it is hardly possible that the advantages mentioned will compensate for the great disadvantages of this method of sustentation. Such instruments are complicated and cumbersome, and involve interference with locomotion and the troublesome necessity of frequent readjustments.

The objections to every form of mechanical support are radical, and admit of no complete removal. Supports do nothing, or next to nothing, toward removing the cause of the difficulty they are expected to meet, even when the results of their use are most satisfactory and complete. Any mode of treatment which shall succeed in restoring the natural supports renders these mechanical substitutes not only unnecessary, but demonstrates their inappropriateness.

The advocates for artificial mechanical sustentation think they find an argument for its use in the assumed analogy between this form of support and those called in requisition by defective limbs. This analogy will not, however, bear close investigation. The limbs are taxed with supporting the body. The uterus has no parallel function, but is itself supported. Another statement frequently made is, that the supporting muscles, being weak, need mechanical aid to supplement their defective function. While the supporting muscles are inadequate, it by no means follows that an artificial substitute for their function will increase their action and power. The reverse is generally conceded to be the case respecting muscles located elsewhere. When it shall be conclusively proved that by enforced inertia, whether by bandaging or removing incentives to contraction, the muscles shall thereby receive more blood, become more contractile and active, then it may be admitted, and not till then, that the arguments and conclusions regarding the enfeebling effects of supporters may be reversed.

IX.

LOCAL APPLICATIONS IN UTERINE DISEASE.

PAIN, wherever located, engages the mental faculties in proportion to its severity. The powers of mind appear to be subordinate to suffering, and nervous action is concentrated at its principal seat. If the seat of pain be beyond the reach of vision, and there be a degree of mystery connected with it, as in case of the pelvic organs, another element, that of imagination, comes in to increase the difficulty. The uterus becomes the focus of thought as well as the seat of feeling, and the suffering woman's ideas of the relations of cause and effect are liable to become inverted. Hence it is that she often regards the contents of the pelvis as the offending as well as the suffering part, and the malaise she feels throughout the system as the consequence, instead of the cause, of her miseries. Indeed, much elucidation of the actually existing relations is required before an invalid thus suffering is convinced that it is not the generative intestine that causes all her ill health, and that what she deems her primary complaint is only secondary, and quite dependent on causes outside the pelvic cavity. Uterine diseases are mainly derived through the same channels as uterine health, viz., through the connection of these parts with the general system.

The erroneous conclusions referred to, as to the origin of pelvic diseases, are not unfrequently countenanced by physicians. This is done by giving preference to local applications of remedies, as though the causes of disease existed mainly in the pelvis, and independent of exterior conditions.

Another circumstance has induced frequent resort to local remedies, until these have come to be considered not only necessary but paramount, viz., the facility with which the vaginal walls, uterine os and neck are reached, examined and medicated through the vagina. While thus remedying what he sees, feels and knows, the physician is naturally indisposed to divide his attention with parts less tangible and definite. These causes cöoperate in withdrawing his mind from the ultimate sources of these diseased manifestations, and to direct attention to effects so easily observed and so readily medicated. So it happens that the absolute and radical causes of disease, consisting of those serious impediments to the local circulation and nutrition heretofore described, have been allowed to remain quite unsuspected. Pelvic nutrition gradually becomes impaired and perverted, and morbid matters accumulate in the obstructed region through causes operating at a distance. Thus the real disease to which we administer is the process which leads to the results already named; the effects disappear only when their causes are removed.

The local remedies referred to are not to be regarded as inappropriate, so much as insufficient. They are effective for only that portion of the disease which consists of consequences or effects, while they are quite irrelevant to this deeper-seated portion, of whose existence we are equally certain, and on which these effects depend. The salutary consequences of these local applications are too limited and circumscribed to meet all the necessities and indications of the case. The really appropriate treatment does not conceal or overlook any actual conditions, but ranges them in their proper order, according to relative importance, giving each and all due place and attention. It includes those belonging to the pelvic organs, and is also careful not to exclude those on which the welfare of the pelvic contents immediately depends.

We will now briefly examine the nature of leading remedial local applications, their relations to vital tissue, and to the system at large, in order to understand their utility in comparison with the treatment which aims primarily at the causes of the diseases under consideration.

Local depletion is the prominent purpose and leading idea of these applications. The most direct agencies are called into requisition. Scarification and leeches are often applied to the mouth of the uterus. Is this way a portion of the blood contained in the part is removed from the over charged tissues. So far, the effect is desirable; but the blood is also removed from the system, an effect undesirable and needless.

Another more frequent mode of diminishing the amount of fluid in the uterine region is by means of caustics. These are a class of substances of decided chemical power. They unite with and thus destroy organized substance, even though vitalized. True medicaments direct vitality; these subvert it. They disorganize the surface, and even the deeper tissues to the extent of their chemical power. Then the serous portion of the contained fluids, being no longer restrained by containing walls, exude from the parenchyma and vessels thus exposed, and pass into the vaginal outlet. The materials commonly employed for this purpose are nitrate of silver, acid nitrate of mercury, nitric acid, chromic acid, permanganate of potassa, potassa fusa, the sulphates of iron, and other materials whose contact with vital tissue causes its destruction. The caustic substance unites with the organic that it comes in contact with, till its causticity is neutralized. The compounds thus formed are supposed to be discharged through the outlet. There is, however, in many cases, very strong evidence that some portion of the medicament is absorbed. This evidence consists in the specific pathological consequences which follow these applications, in cases where they have been many times repeated.

These applications are made to the vaginal walls, the uterine os, cervical canal, and often to the lining of the cavity. From the list of caustic substances the physician selects according as the different articles are deemed by him to be most appropriate to the condition in which he finds the different portions of the generative intestine.

A caustic application is not presumed to have a strictly curative effect. When its avidity for organized substances becomes neutralized its direct action ceases, and it becomes comparatively inoffensive. Its function is theoretically to remove degenerative and offensive animal matter, and thereby prevent the unfavorable influence of decaying organic material upon contiguous vital tissues. A local ulceration is thus virtually converted into a fresh wound, with active healing tendencies. This is the most favorable view of the effects; but caustics are by no means indispensable for this end. There are innocuous materials which serve the purpose even better. But to prevent the production of local, morbid material supersedes the need of the employment of either and is obviously the better way.

Another is, however, the chief effect desired of caustic appliances; and this is to relieve the overburdened vessels and the interstitial parts of their painful tension, by exudation of a portion of their contents, causing the capillaries to contract. The normal condition of these parts is thus approximated. The grateful sense of relief which follows appears to justify the means, especially in the absence of a knowledge of more complete and permanent remedial applications.

But most forms of disease of the uterus and its connections, having their basis in local hyperæmia, are possible only in consequence of a greater facility of flow of fluids into, than out of, these organs. It is evident that the local applications can have but little if any influence on this fact. The correction of the circulation in this particular can be effected only through the active agency of parts outside the pelvis. These parts and the general muscular system must be made to receive and retain more blood, so as to prevent its accumulation in the pelvis. A perpetual, unchecked onflow to the pelvis quite counteracts the benefit hoped from local depletion. The pelvic capillaries immediately become re-distended as before, in the absence of precautionary means.

Practically, it has been found that the improvement procured by caustics is maintained only through their repeated application, at such intervals as experience in individual cases may dictate. It would hence appear that such improvement is not real, but simulative and temporary. It will also be observed that the supposed benefit thus derived is indirect and secondary, a consequence of the vital endeavor to repair recent injuries, while the direct effect is destructive.

Drugs of another class employed in local medication of the pelvic contents represent an inferior degree of chemical power. They are incapable of destroying the surface to which they are applied. They form a series, and include those which produce stimulative, astringent, alterative and tonic effects, and in these and probably other ways, not well understood, modify local nutrition. Some portion of drugs thus applied is doubtless absorbed, and produces effects not confined to the pelvis. An outflow of serous fluid into the vaginal cavity is produced by some of these applications; in other cases the circulation is accelerated, whereby the capillary contents are diminished. The medical agencies thus used are numerous and varied in their chemical nature and physiological relationship.

The abundant resources furnished by drugs have not, I conceive, been sufficiently examined with reference to application in uterine affections.

Physicians, have been too eager to secure decided immediate effects to investigate patiently the claims of remedies which they conceive to be slower in their effects, overlooking the fact that these latter are in general of a permanent and reliable character. It has been in my way to experiment much in the direction now indicated, and experience has led me to displace many of the remedies in popular repute by others combining mildness with superior permanent efficacy.

It is a serious mistake to suppose that applications which represent the greatest chemical power, such as caustics, therefore embody the most healing or curative efficacy. The true medicament simply supplements the vital endeavor, and renders it more complete and perfect.

Too much, however, should not be expected of even the most appropriate applications. Their proper sphere is limited to local and transient purposes—helps to the radical and curative means which it is my purpose to set forth. These aids may be employed as such, but not with the idea that the cure depends thereon.

A third class of remedies used in the local treatment of pelvic disease consists in the topical application of those sedative drugs also administered in the ordinary way.

A curative effect is hardly expected of this class of applications. Their function is more that of diminishing the consciousness of the pathological state than of removing it; but the use of this class of remedies, locally, is no doubt justified in certain invalids whose physiological state is much under the control of the sensations and emotions. The influence of such remedies is attainable only by local absorption of some portion of the drug.

There may be emergencies when the physician may even be thankful for the aid this class of medicaments can afford, but he should be cautious about favoring them with his prolonged confidence. Whatever advantage may temporarily accrue to the local nerves, the general effect of sedative drugs on the system must be admitted to be any thing but desirable.

The reader will bear in mind that cases requiring interference strictly surgical are not at present under consideration.

The usual practice in uterine cases has now

been very briefly commented upon. It admits of an endless variety of detail and modification, according to the views of different physicians, respecting the nature of the local affection and the estimate they may place upon remedies.

It is not my purpose to condemn. Current medical literature and practice represents the best thought in its various departments, and is entitled to all respect. But few of its data are absolute in their nature, and it is more progressive than most of the sciences. It has not grown more by accretion than by succession of ideas. Everything is good in its time and place. The rational inference is, that still more advanced ideas and methods will, in due time, render the present of little account. The *good*, gracefully but inevitably, yields to *better*, whenever the latter becomes apparent.

The purpose of this work the reader can hardly fail to understand. It is simply to exhibit the reasons and evidences on which rest my convictions, confirmed by long experience and abundant opportunities, that current medical practice *is not based*, as it should be, *on the most important facts* of pelvic pathology, Such practice seems to ignore the most essential, the most vital point. It takes little or no practical account of the *causes* of pelvic hyperæmia, out of which, in general, the various common forms of pelvic disease must, of necessity, proceed. Failure to recognize these causes is equivalent to a limitation of legitimate remedial resources, and contentment with temporary and inconsequential expedients.

The direct proof of the correctness of the principles set forth in these pages is easily attained. Pelvic hyperæmia will be seen to disappear on putting these principles into practical operation. But this is far from being all. The *diseases* which are products and outgrowths of this condition will be shown to disappear with, generally, a very gratifying degree of readiness. The successful treatment of invalids by radical methods is by no means confined to the incipient stages of pelvic disease. On the contrary, the power of the methods now to be detailed is confirmed by their success in the most difficult and trying cases, if non-malignant in character. Let it be understood that the best results may be attained *without* the use of topical medication of any kind whatever. I state this to show the radical and potential nature of the remedial measures proposed, but do not say that topical aid would not, in many cases, add to the rapidity of restoration.

It is proper also to say that there are other considerations than those of strict scientific propriety which will often dictate the kind of remedies to be employed, and which will quite frequently justify the use of means not absolutely relevant to the case. Female education is to be taken into due account, and female expectations respected, or the physician will find in the nervous condition and in the mental habit of his patient an irremovable barrier to the success of his best remedies. Physicians often observe that chronic illnesses are treated with indifferent success, unless the mind and feelings accord with the remedial means employed.

While, then, it is my purpose to bring to view old but neglected facts, and to invoke from them a *new* experience and practice, rather than to condemn what is established and justified, it becomes my duty to point out some of the shortcomings of the essentially local method of applying remedies, and the disadvantages arising therefrom:

1. The first of these has already received attention, and consists in the fact that local ap-

plications *have no control whatever over what is demonstrably the usual, and certainly the most potent, cause of pelvic affections.* It is plain that the uterine circulation is not permanently aided in any considerable degree, nor is the superincumbent weight removed, by any form of local medication; and, so far as pelvic disease depends on pelvic hyperæmia, the usual and most potent causes for its continuance are quite as operative *with* as without the treatment referred to. The local applications may transiently remove the existing condition, but are of little or no account in securing permanency of this effect.

2. We have seen that depletive local applications to the womb remove its congestion and inflammation partly, perhaps by exciting an exudation from the part overburdened with serous fluids. The loss of such fluids, rich in albumen, may not appreciably affect the general health. We are not conscious of the minor circumstances which affect our power. But there can be no doubt, as before stated, that an active local outlet for fluids causes those of the general system to *set* in the direction of the drain, thus refilling and soon redistending the part. In this way the previous hyperæmic condition is nearly,

sometimes fully, restored. While but little progress is thus made toward a cure, the system becomes habituated to an unwholesome reaction. This is the explanation of the need of frequent repetitions of such applications in order to maintain the relief first experienced. The *real* advantage secured is simply that of change of nutritive fluid, and consequent improved nutrition in the overburdened and sluggish parts—an object far better accomplished by other means, capable, perhaps, of producing less rapid effects, but more certain cures.

3. Frequently repeated applications of strong medicaments to the womb tend to the production of a morbid state of the nerves of the pelvic region, and through these the whole nervous system. This conclusion is justified by comparison of cases treated chiefly by the local measures already specified, with similar cases treated without recourse to these remedies. It is well known that this class of invalids is subject to severe nervous troubles, such as persistent pain in the loins, back, legs, as well as pelvis, and in great disproportion to the local disease to which its origin is referred. These pains often appear even to increase with the

progress of treatment, spite of the persistent sedative and antiphlogistic applications to which the pelvic organs are subjected. This aggravation of symptoms and persistence of pain is entirely consonant with the supposition stated.

These effects, or at least some of them, not unfrequently appear in consequence of so simple an application as that of drenching the vagina with the cold water douche, so frequently recommended. While this operation primarily reduces the temperature and imparts a tonic, contractile condition to the pelvic region, it does not end with these effects. A reaction toward the pelvis is apt to be superinduced, resulting in an increased supply of blood, increase of heat, and of all the conditions of exaggerated sensibility, thus making the pelvis a centre of both mental and organic influences, which easily glide into a permanent morbid condition.

The presumption of injury to the nerves by indiscreet or even by ordinary topical treatment is amply justified by rational considerations. For, though the pelvic region has no superior endowment of common sensibility, yet we know that the functions of this region are second in importance to none in the system, and that they have most profound and extensive sympathies. The generative system is indeed a great centre of nervous power. The inference is at least plausible that morbid sensory impressions—such as are necessarily made by the application of the more potent substances named, and even by the sedative class of remedies, which are supposed to affiliate in some way with nerve substance—should produce an effect by no means confined to the pelvic region, but be radiated more or less extensively throughout the nervous system. My opportunities for observation have acquainted me with numerous instances of this class of invalids, whose prolonged disease has rendered them well nigh hopeless as well as helpless, and whose continued suffering I have been constrained to refer, in good part, to unnecessary and misdirected remedial efforts, especially those directed to the local symptoms, while the real cause suffered neglect.

Invalids of this class are, in general, much more difficult of cure than cases that have not been overmuch tampered with by local remedies. This shows that nerve disease has been superadded to that of other tissues. It is well known that nerve substance recovers much more slowly from injuries, however inflicted, than any other form of living tissue.

Any continued and peculiar aberration in nervous power is evidence of loss of integrity of the nervous substance. The forms which nervous disease, thus superinduced, are most liable to take are local and general neuralgia and perverted and exaggerated sensibility. These forms of nervous affection not unfrequently extend to the cerebro-spinal system, so as to produce irrepressible emotional activity. Certainly such consequences should greatly detract from the estimate placed upon the use of local applications for the cure of disease having its origin at points remote from its manifestation.

4. The connection of mind and thought with pelvic disorders has been referred to. This power is forcibly directed by the senses, and is susceptible of becoming permanently fixed upon any interior organ. The effect is highly injurious. The most potent means of perverting functional activity, and of causing it to degenerate, is thus set in action. Illustrations of this fact are not confined to cases of pelvic disease, but are familiar and striking as applied to other parts of the body. All physicians have seen the effect,

on the health of the stomach, for example, of constant watchfulness of that organ. The nutritive condition of the abdomen, head, or indeed any important physiological centre, is liable in some temperaments to perversion from the same cause.

The uterus and appendages are ordained by nature to be the centre of peculiar physiological interest. The unfathomable mysteries of procreation and the perpetuity of the species are involved therein. These organs are also in some way related to the deepest and most permanent feelings of the heart. In proportion as these matters transcend knowledge do they furnish food for the imagination, and in the pathological states growing out of hyperæmia the effect is peculiarly retroactive and morbid, and constantly operating to increase and aggravate the disease. The effect of calling the attention to the pelvic region so strongly as is done by means of frequent local applications must therefore be to increase this kind of morbid action, and to fix and perpetuate the disease.

5. Closely connected with these consequences of prolonged local treatment for pelvic disease is the occasional contraction of a morbid habit of

being thus treated; it might almost be said, a fondness for it. Of the fact of the possible formation of such a habit on the part of certain females, most physicians who treat this class of cases are able to testify. This is striking evidence of the correctness of the principles asserted above; that local medication is capable of causing derangement of the nerves of the whole system, extending these irregularities to the emotional nature.

These are some of the consequences of local uterine treatment, and are inevitable if such treatment be made excessive and exclusive for a prolonged period; in other words, these are the frequent results of the *abuse* of it. But, because I insist that such treatment is so commonly misused, the reader will not understand me as *discarding* local applications in pelvic diseases. My chief object has been to show that by using mere local treatment the essential disease itself is left neglected, untouched, and even unsought; that symptoms only command the attention, and symptoms that will certainly subside and become of trifling account whenever the essential malady is recognized and properly provided for.

Physicians whose resources in the treatment

of uterine disease are mainly limited to the employment of local applications, are by no means agreed as to the kind of effect such medication produces, or its value. Dr. E. R. Peaslee, in an exhaustive article* on *Intra-uterine Medication*, comes to this conclusion:—"Endometrial applications should be but very rarely resorted to by the gynecologist; being proper *only* in case of metorrhœa (uterine catarrh) and metorrhagia, (acute bleeding,) and perhaps sometimes in chronic endometritis without a discharge." He further says that "they are often used in conditions not at all justifying them;" "that they have thus far produced, on the whole, more evil than good." He therefore recommends, as a substitute for other intra-uterine medication, what he calls *endometrial ingestion*, consisting of medicated ointments, applied by means of a probe, the end of which is wrapped in cotton. In view of the abundant mucous discharge usually provoked when these parts are thus touched, washing away any adhering medicament, this mode of medication would seem to be innocuous enough.

* New York Medical Journal, Ju'y, 1870.

Dr. Thomas* says:—"The fact is notorious that the local treatment of these diseases is not as successful in its results as we could wish." "The treatment may extend over months, perhaps over years, before a cure is effected." Again, "Every one who has had experience in the treatment of these disorders must have been struck with surprise at the wonderful improvement exerted on cases *which have long resisted local means*, by a sea voyage, a visit to a watering place, a course of sea-bathing, or a few months passed in the country."

†"My impression is, that intra-uterine injections do not constitute an advance in the treatment of uterine diseases; that they have done, and are going to do, a great deal of harm; and that though now they are popular, their evil results will cause them, after a more thorough trial, to be discarded." Again, "My own impression is, that where intra-uterine injection is practised, a certain number of cases will die, from penetration of the fluid through the fallopian tubes." "I see no *necessity* for intra-uterine injections."

* On Diseases of Women. By T. Gaillard Thomas, M.D.

† Extracts from remarks by Dr. Thomas before the Medical Society of the County of New York, May 23, 1870.

Dr. George T. Elliot, president at a late stated meeting of the New York County Medical Society, the subject of Uterine Therapeutics being under discussion, as reported in the "Record," remarked that—

"He was profoundly convinced that one of the most important elements of success in solving the difficult problem of the treatment of diseases of women consisted in securing such a mode of life as would compel muscular activity, and so equalize the circulation. For many patients he was in the habit of ordering localized movements, &c., until they were able to take out-of-door exercise. In a large class of cases of anæmia and amenorrhœa, where the patient complained of weakness, wanting to keep in the house and loll on the sofa, he had more confidence in this physiological mode of treatment than in all others. *If this were properly carried out, the local treatment now so much in vogue, and the ever ready resort to the speculum, might commonly be dispensed with.*"

"The sentiment appears to be gaining ground," to use the words of a speaker at one of the meetings of the Medical Society, "that in all cases of very troublesome intra-uterine affection there is some constitutional dyscrasy; and that no topical treatment can be of any permanent avail, without keeping this in mind and giving the most careful attention to constitutional treatment and hygienic measures." The expression of sentiments like the above by the leading gynecologists of the day, betokens a tendency to reaction from the weakly dependence on local medication which has for many years characterized current practice. These methods have been consequent upon the invention of facilities for the employment of that style of medication, but cannot be sustained against broader and more comprehensive views of pathology.

The over-confidence with which some women regard their medical advisers on the one hand, and the over-estimate which some physicians place upon local treatment on the other, is thus described by the senior editor of the Pacific Medical and Surgical Journal:

"Now let us come home and bring to judgment a sin in the family. Within the profession there is a species of quackery which is advertised not by the printing press, but by the uterine speculum. There prevails very extensively among our women a singular disorder of which the most prominent symptom is a passion for uterine exploration. To some extent, medical practitioners are responsible for the general prevalence of this malady. It is easy for sensitive females to persuade themselves that their afflictions, from the toothache downward, are due to falling of the womb, or ulcerations, or tumors; and he is the sharpest doctor who first detects the difficulty. Here comes in the charlatan, to exaggerate the disease if there be any, and to beguile the patient with promises of cure. Henceforth the speculum becomes to the poor woman an essential part of the routine of life. Caustic, the knife, and various manipulations look like work; and she is charmed with the industrious and energetic attentions of the professional mechanic. By and by the bubble bursts, and for all the good that has been done by subjecting the uterus to a course of torture, its proprietor might as well have adopted the treatment accredited to that miracle of scientific skill, Li-potai, namely, the application of a blister to the crown of the head, to raise the fallen womb to its place."

"It is to be hoped that the fashion of women to have recourse to local treatment has passed to its culmination, and with it the professional mania for persecuting that organ. The highest authorities have taken the back course, and condemn their own uterine surgery in some respects. We may therefore indulge reasonable expectations that this form of treatment will henceforth be limited to its legitimate and restricted sphere."

Considering the physician's anxious and weary endeavors for the good of his patient, she has in general no right to interpose objections to his measures, so long as these are useful. But she has a right to so much knowledge in these matters which so vitally concern her as will enable her to form an intelligent judgment. Her disease, it is more than probable, was acquired in ignorance of the physiological principles which, if observed, would have led to prevention. But having become the subject of disease, she is compelled to select the class of remedial measures she shall employ; there is no evading this necessity. The alternatives may be presented as follows:

Whether to employ remedies, the nature and effect of which the patient has not the remotest idea; to be subjected to frequent, often useless, sometimes purposeless, local examinations; to endure the torture of the sensitive feelings natural to one jealous of the maintenance of her highest womanhood; to endure the applications to internal organs of the most powerfully destructive chemicals which science has invented; to be left liable to anomalous affections of the pelvic region and perhaps of the whole system as the secondary effect of remedial applications; to suffer actual repression of so much vitality as is represented in the sustaining muscles, and to suffer the liability to pulmonary and digestive diseases as a consequence; and lastly, to endure disease, acquired in ignorance, without any effort toward the removal of those conditions whose continued operation is sure to perpetuate it, on the one hand, or the principles and methods I have herein presented, on the other. Between these the difficulty of choosing must gradually diminish, in proportion as their real nature and value become subjects of intelligent reflection and inquiry. The mind naturally prefers the least equivocal, the most simple and direct.

X.

FURTHER STATEMENTS OF PRINCIPLES AVAILABLE IN PELVIC THERAPEUTICS.

A LEADING purpose of the body is manifestly to evolve force,—the force employed to overcome its own inertia, and the resistance of external objects. This latter purpose is under the guidance of the intelligence and will, which are also modifications of force. The capacity of the body to completely secure these ends is, in general, the measure of its health.

The manifestation of force in an animal organism appears to represent the collective energy of myriads of interior, invisible, elemental parts. The expression of motion by muscular acts is the aggregated and directed action of the minutest muscular elements. The generalized views of modern authorities on this subject probably approximate this statement. The chemical products incessantly passing from the body are the evidences of chemical changes within it. These chemical changes represent organic disintegration. This latter act, for which facilities are afforded in the constant motion of fluids, and the consequent renewed contact of constituent elements, relieves and sets free the force previously embodied in organization, and necessary to the constitution of the primary organic molecule or form. This force hence becomes an available emanation of animal bodies.

Precedent to this, however, is organic growth, or composition, effected by mere solution and arrangement of the atomic elements of organized substance, without disturbing its combining force.

All these primary actions, chemical and organic, of various kinds, are included under the general term, nutrition. This implies both the formation and dissolution of organized matter. Composition and decomposition, growth and destruction, are necessarily coincident, and interdependent. The powers manifested by nerves and muscles are the ultimate consequences of these nutritive actions. The details and proofs of these statements constitute the science of physiology.

It is the evident purpose of medical treatment to acquire control over these elemental acts, from which alone all power emanates; for there is no other channel through which health can be influenced.

There are probably many legitimate methods for acquiring this control in some degree, which may be employed in the same forms of disease, because there are many ways of exciting chemical and organic disturbance and activity. Among these, physicians exercise their preference according to their knowledge.

The reader, in tracing with us the origin of disease in the class of invalids under consideration, has found it to lie in certain specific defects. These may be said to consist of defective power and motion in the muscles controlling respiration, and defective power and tone in the capillaries of the pelvic viscera. These defects give rise to others, specific in location and in mode of manifestation, and ordinarily regarded as *the* disease, without going further back.

In other words, pathological symptoms appearing in the pelvic region denote defective nutrition and activity in those superior organs which dominate the position and circulation of the contents of the pelvis. To perfect the nutrition of these dominant parts is therefore equivalent to the sustaining of the visceral weight, the removal of capillary obstructions, the interchange of capillary with contiguous interstitial fluids, and the return of these organs to their normal condition from their periodical functional hyperæmia. The remedy most needed to secure a return from a pathological to a physiological condition is that which increases the nutrition of the parts so suffering.

We have seen that local remedies produce this effect only to a very limited and imperfect extent. The obvious reason is that particular parts of the body are dependent upon other parts and the general system, and are not self-sustained, as the practice of local remedies implies. The vitality of every part of the body is maintained through conditions at a distance from it, and apparently in no wise directly connected with it. The body is a whole, and the recovery of parts that have become disordered can be compassed only by invigorating and increasing the vital energy of the whole system. This is the inflexible condition of bodily recovery, health and power, from which there can be no safe departure; and without compliance with this condition, there can be no certain or permanent cure of disorders that seem local only because the unpracticed eye fails to detect the subtle connection of part with part, and the dependence of each organ upon the vigor and soundness of the entire system.

The system evolves force in all its minutest power-evolving departments. It remains to be shown that this power is susceptible of conduction and transfer; and that special localities, where it is deficient, may easily be made the recipient of that which has its origin in the system at large. This principle is applied whenever we exert muscular power; for though in case of a special act the muscles of the acting part directly afford the power exerted, yet the conditions for its continuance are coincidently transferred from parts quite beyond that of its exercise—from the whole system. Besides, the nerve power which excites and instigates muscular contraction is itself a result of actions quite distant and distinct from the locality of its manifestation. This energy as well as the due supply of material are therefore transferred in every manifestation of force. It follows that the aggregate powers of the system may be regarded as a reservoir of force, capable of being called in any direction.

In this view we contemplate on the one hand *force needed;* on the other *force supplied.* These are the two terms of the vital equation which our system regards as theoretically complimental and equal. When considered in connection with pathology, the equivalent forms of expression are, *disease; remedy.*

This force may be self-generated, or, to a limited extent, derived. I desire to show that the process of generation may be augmented, to respond to specific needs; also to demonstrate that, in default of systemic force, these interior motions on which force depends can be excited by exterior means—by the application of exterior and ordinary force, in such a way that the organic element may be able with facility to appropriate force, whereby it becomes auxiliary to the intrinsic molecular motions. In this way force becomes remedial.

Medical science is teeming with devices, almost always in the form of drugs, and hence chemical in their aspect, nature and workings, for the purpose of stimulating these nutritive actions in local parts as well as in the general system. None, however, can attain to the degree and the purity of effect of MOTION itself. None are so energetic, none so localized, none so economical of vitality. This agent excites fully and only those minute, chemical and molecular actions by which vital energy is evolved. By other agencies, we know not what irrelevant actions are superinduced, and what expenditure of vital power is caused.

Motion may, therefore, properly be prescribed and employed to restore the nutritive conditions necessary to increase the generation of power and to localize such power in deficient parts.

In health, the actions on which it depends are chiefly instigated by the will. In disease, the incentive needs to be supplied from other sources. The action of the will is at once difficult and injurious. Hence these actions are usually excited and controlled by medicines. In chronic cases this method is simply unnecessary, often injurious. Motion can always be communicated to interior parts, direct and without chemical intervention; and the action can be derived from exterior causes, especially by the employment of exterior common force.

It is hence seen that in two ways exercise becomes remedial. One is by *active motion*, when the muscles are caused to act through the will; the other is by *passive motion*, in which a limited portion or region of the body is rendered physiologically active, by mechanical causes.

Such exercises or motions, prescribed with strict reference to definite therapeutic effects, have received the appellation of MOVEMENTS.

The special use of active movements is to give direction to the powers and resources of the system, through a particular channel to a designated location, so as to supply it in a higher degree with the conditions of vital energy. The whole system is thus caused to contribute to and perfect the vital power of a limited portion.

*Passive Movements** are employed to produce a variety of therapeutic effects, many of which are otherwise difficult of attainment. They may be so used as:

To renew and refresh the circulation and therefore the nutrition of any selected local point.

To cause the blood to flow in increased amount from any designated part.

To cause the blood to flow in increased amount toward a given part.

To cause interstitial local absorption, and the reduction of œdematous and other swellings.

* For a more complete account of Passive Vibratory Movements, their mode of application, and their effects, the reader is referred to an article by the author in the New York Medical Journal for November, 1869.

To cause contraction of capillary vessels, previously distended.

To secure relief from pain.

To correct and perfect the products of waste passing from the body.

To increase the use of oxygen by the system.

To supersede other means for securing local depletion, counter-irritation, and revulsion.

In chronic diseases, the modification of the quality of nutrition commensurate with the needs of the case may be effected by increased use of oxygen by the system. Various drugs produce this effect to a moderate degree, and for only a transient period; but in this class of cases, the results thus fitfully obtained are of comparatively trifling account. The failure of the respiratory muscles, which always must precede and attend pelvic difficulties, also implies deficient use of oxygen, and the consequent accumulation of insufficiently oxidized wasting products.

Vibratory and other passive movements, precede and coöperate with the development of the mechanical conditions for health. Both are indispensable to attain the purposes in view.

MECHANICAL INVENTIONS IN AID OF REMEDIAL TREATMENT.

The advantages derived by the well from exercise has always been coveted for invalids, and endeavors without number have been made to render such advantages in some way available. These attempts however, have been at best but partially successful. This is because the methods adopted have generally involved a harmful expenditure of the invalid's own power. It has not been seen with sufficient clearness that, since the capacity for the self-regeneration of power is wanting in invalids, that which is needed to carry forward the physiological processes must be derived from some abundant exterior source. The idea of force supplied has, indeed, been a good deal experimented with, but only through the instrumentality of the hands of an assistant, nurse, or operator, who applies sundry rubbings, stretchings and manipulatings of a heterogeneous character, and controlled by no very definite purpose.

However plausible the theory of aid so applied may appear, no very decided or reliable advantage can be thus gained for the invalid. The power of the assistant is too irregular, unintelligent, and insufficiently controlled by the invalid and too soon exhausted to be depended on. This source of power, the hand, may at times be very desirable as supplementary to other sources, but it never has acquired, and never can, the distinction of a far-reaching and universal remedy. Foot travel would as soon supersede steam conveyance for long distances.

The desideratum in this case is power abundant and controllable. Fortunately, the universe is replete with force, ready for human service. It is quite unnecessary to depend on the fitful and limited supply an assistant is capable of affording. There has only been wanting mechanical adaptations suitable to give it direction.

Feeling the imperative need in my practice of power auxiliary to that supplied by the hand, in carrying these ideas into effect—the positive demand for more efficacious, constant, and reliable power, and knowing no methods adapted or designed to secure this end, I have been compelled to invent certain instruments by which force is employed for curative purposes.

These instruments are simply the conduits and regulators of force, derived from whatever source. Gravitation serves to operate some of these instruments. In this case, the gravitating force of the invalid or of an assistant, or of an oscillating weight, is transferred by the instrument to some selected portion of the invalid's body.

But great achievements of force applied remedially are secured only when it proceeds from some constant and abundant source, as that derived from steam. It can then be so directed and controlled by these instruments as to respond to the indications of chronic disease. The employment of these mechanical devices has been attended by the most marked and gratifying success, far exceeding that attainable by the hands of assistants; and serving a variety of other purposes than those which come within the scope of ordinary remedies. Some of the instruments used in the special class of cases treated of in this work will be described in the succeeding pages.

XI.

MEANS OF SECURING SUSTENTATION OF THE PELVIC CONTENTS. EXAMPLES OF MOVEMENTS.

An important feature of remedial treatment for difficulties referable to the pelvis, is the elevation of its contents, and their maintenance in this improved position. This result may be perfectly accomplished by causes acting above the pelvis, but not below it. All efforts acting in the latter direction are necessarily failures, more or less signal, because all such means are without the least influence, either in removing the superincumbent weight, or in restoring the lost motions to these parts. Such means can, at most, only resist the weight, not remove it, and will prevent rather than aid the natural motions.

The first thing in furtherance of the end proposed is plainly to provide room higher in the cavity of the trunk to which the pelvic contents can rise. This can be done only by increasing the space at the upper portion of this cavity.

The whole visceral mass must rise to occupy the space the moment it is provided. No vacuum can exist.

The body is abundantly provided by nature with the means for maintaining the adjustments of its parts. In health the means for elevating and sustaining the abdominal and pelvic contents are in effective action; in disease these means fail. With a little knowledge and due attention to the defect involved, they may be put in effective operation and the suffering parts fully relieved.

These means or conditions consist in the mobility of the walls of the chest, and particularly that portion formed by the diaphragm. The restoration of power and action to the muscles which cause motion of the chest-walls is the first step in the fulfillment of the proposed object. In order to enable the chest muscles to effect the utmost distention of the chest-walls, it is necessary that their upper extremities be fixed above their usual position. This is easily done by raising the arms, for the predominant muscles of the outer walls of the chest are attached by their superior extremities to the upper bone of the arms. If these muscles be made to act, while their upper ends are thus fixed by this upward position of the arms, the lower border of the ribs is made to move upward and outward. The entire walls of the chest participate in the same motion, diminishing in degree toward its upper portion.

The mechanical result of all such movements is to increase the space between the ribs, elevate the diaphragm, and therefore to increase the amount of space below the diaphragm. Following are examples of exercise producing this effect in the highest degree.

1. *MOVEMENT OR PROCESS FOR INCREASING THE SPACE IN THE SUPERIOR PORTION OF THE CAVITY OF THE TRUNK.*

The patient assumes the horizontal position, with back resting on a couch, the arms stretched upward, parallel with the body and each other.

An assistant, standing in a convenient position near the head of the patient, grasps each of her hands and makes gentle resistance while she slowly raises the arms to the perpendicular position and nearly at right angles with the trunk. The resistance must be nicely proportioned to the strength of the patient, not enough to task it unduly, yet sufficient to stimulate vigorously its production. The assistant, by gentle pressure upon the hands of the patient, now slowly returns the arms to the commencing position. This action may be repeated four or five times, the assistant accurately gauging the patient's strength, and adjusting the resistance to the increased power the patient affords at each successive endeavor.

In this movement the arms are levers, which act through certain connecting muscles upon the chest. The principal muscles of the anterior portion of the chest, the pectorals, are distributed over and attached by one extremity of their fibres to the ribs; the other extremity of these fibres converge and form a strong tendon attached to the upper portion of the bone of the arm.

The action of these muscles in the position described is expended upon the ribs. The intercostal muscles participate in the same action, producing the effect of raising the anterior ends of the ribs, spreading them apart and increasing the intervening space. This action expands the diaphragm, increases the circumference at the base of the chest and the amount of space immediately below it. Toward the space thus provided, the contents of the abdomen at once move, diminishing the circumference at the lower portion of the abdomen, and withdrawing the pressure of its contents from the pelvis. If the patient be very weak, this process should be applied to one side first, and afterward to the other.

Following is a modification of the above, to be executed by patients, when not too feeble, without an assistant.

2 *SIMILAR PROCESS FOR THE SAME PURPOSE, EXECUTED WITHOUT ASSISTANCE.*

The position is the same as above, except that the hands grasp a small weight of from one half to two pounds, according to the strength.

The arms move slowly in the plane of the body, describing parts of circles, of which the shoulders are the centres, till they reach the sides of the body. They then slowly return, travelling in the opposite direction, through the same space, till they again meet above the head. This action may be repeated three or four times.

In this, as in the preceding movement, the arms are levers, through which the gravitation of the weights take the place of the efforts of the assistant, in acting upon the anterior portion of the chest. The separation of the ribs, the distention of the diaphragm, the drawing upward of the whole abdominal contents, and the relief of the contents of the pelvis from the effects of pressure, are all similar to those produced by No. 1.

3. *MOVEMENT FOR RAISING THE ABDOMINAL AND PELVIC CONTENTS THROUGH ACTION OF THE CHEST, BY APPARATUS.*

A very effective mode of accomplishing this purpose is by the apparatus whose description follows.

A post is so contrived in bi-lateral parts that one part will easily glide upon the other, and can be readily fixed at any desired point. The top of the post can thus be adjusted to the shoulders of persons of different heights. To the top of the post is affixed an axle, from which rises a lever provided with a handle. The lever may also be lengthened to suit the length of the arms. A pendulum, bearing a weight, is connected with the axle by a ratchet. By means of the ratchet, the position of the pendulum, and therefore the leverage and force with which the weight acts upon the person, can easily be controlled. A well-padded bar projects from the upper end of the post, at the same side as the projecting handle.

Having adjusted the padded bar to the proper height, which is at the lower portion of the shoulder-blades, the sliding handle to the length of the arms when fully extended, and the weighted pendulum so as to afford the proper degree of resistance, which should be nicely proportioned to the strength, the patient places her back in contact with the bar and grasps the handle, while standing firmly on her feet. For ordinary use, the lever and pendulum should be in nearly a straight line: if there be deformity, or contracted muscles, or great weakness, the handle should be inclined forward; if there be a good degree of vigor, it should incline backward, and the force which the weight exerts upon the muscles will be varied accordingly.

The slightest effort of the arms in the position above described causes the weighted pendulum to diverge. The degree of divergence is in exact proportion to such effort. Having reached the maximum of divergence, the weight immediatel becomes a falling body, and reacting, causes the lever, handle, and patient's arms to be pressed strongly back, until arrested by the resistance of the muscles of the chest upon which this action wholly falls. The padded bar supplies the necessary counter pressure to the back, at a point quite below the anterior portion of the chest, which, therefore, receives the action and momentum of the weight.

This motion gives very strong action to all the anterior muscles of the chest, to the diaphragm and the abdominal walls. It causes the chest to become strongly arched forward, raises as well as distends the diaphragm, causes a lifting of the whole of the abdominal and pelvic viscera, and necessarily has great effect in aiding the return or venous circulation throughout the lower portion of the body. The use of this instrument preserves suppleness in the joints connecting the ribs with the spine, and obviates any tendency of the tendons and cartilages of the chest to become inelastic and fixed. It transmits the motions of respiration to the abdominal and to the pelvic viscera, and through this means protects these parts against congestion, and consequently preserves their health.

The patient may present either side instead of the back to the bar, or indeed any other portion of the chest. She will then grasp the handle with one instead of both hands. In this case the whole effect of the process falls upon one side only of the chest. In any case, the use of the instrument serves to expand that portion of the chest upon which the action falls, whether it be the anterior or either lateral half. It develops the strength of any portion receiving the action.

This instrument utilizes the force of gravitation. It applies this force to counteract the gravitation of the contents of the trunk and pelvis. The weight of the pendulum is made to balance that of the organs named, through the levers of the instrument, and the arms of the persons using it. The whole of this force acts through the muscles of the chest and abdomen, and therefore increases their development and power.

The instrument works with the utmost ease. Scarcely more than the weight of the upstretched arms is required to set it in action; it therefore makes but small demand on the will, and does not produce fatigue.

The adjustments of the instrument allow increase of resistance to correspond with the improvement of the strength, to any extent that may be demanded.

4. *MOVEMENT FOR CULTIVATING THE POWER OF THE CHEST, AND INCREASING ITS CONTROL OF THE PARTS BENEATH.*

The invalid lies with the head and shoulders slightly raised, the arms stretched upward, and parallel with the trunk.

An assistant grasps both hands of the patient, and offers gentle resistance, while she slowly draws her arms downward and into close contact with the sides, causing them to become acutely bent at the elbows. This resistance is so supplied as to correspond with the varying degrees of power afforded by the muscles of the patient during the progressive stages of the movement. This power is less at the beginning and termination of the movement, and greater at the intermediate points. The assistant, maintaining his grasp, draws the arms of the patient upward and backward, while the patient slightly resists, till the commencing position is reached. If the patient be quite weak, she need make no effort; this may be left entirely to the assistant, while the muscles and nerves of the patient receive the assistant's power. This form of movement is entirely passive, and should be applied to one side only at a time.

The effects are quite similar to those produced by the previously described operations. On account of the easy, recumbent position in which it is taken, and the manner of its application, this movement is peculiarly agreeable to the feelings, and is noticeably followed by quietude.

Operations of the class now described, adapted to increase the power and size of the chest and the extent of its motions, are of primary importance. They exert an immediate and profound control over the circulation of the pelvic organs. Whether these motions occur spontaneously, as in health, or by design, as in the processes described, their influence is absolutely necessary to the welfare of the contents of the pelvis.

Movements similar to the above may be extemporized to an indefinite extent. It will be sufficient to suggest that all motions of the body, whether bending or twisting, made with the arms fixed upward, by stretching or clasping the hands above the head, produce effects of the same kind. Such operations can be performed without an assistant if there be moderate strength. If an assistant be employed, more varied and more pronounced effects are easily attainable.

The assistant is presumed to know at what points the muscular power of the invalid is defective. At such points the assistant supplies resistance sufficient to excite the efforts and bring out the energies of the patient, which are consequently concentrated at the point thus selected.

The assistant also supplies the energy required when this is deficient in the invalid; so that the effect in the tissues is secured without expenditure on the part of the patient. Such aid, therefore, obviates fatigue, while securing all the advantages derivable from action.

XII.

METHODS OF EMPLOYING GRAVITATION AS AN AID IN RESTORING THE POSITION OF THE PELVIC CONTENTS.

The statement of invalids that their sufferings are due to prolapsus or depression of the uterus, is, in the light of the preceding facts, a confession that the sustaining elements are at fault. Every mundane object is affected by gravitation. It is a common property of all things. The position of objects depends on where this force is just balanced by other forces. The state of rest is the equipoise of antagonistic forces. In the human body this antagonizing or sustaining power, as regards the contents of the abdomen and pelvis, resides chiefly in the muscles of the anterior and central portions of the trunk. The ordinary use of these muscles in all wholesome occupations maintains the supremacy of their power. This, with the rythmic motions of respiration in which they participate, amply serves the purpose of sustaining the contents of the inferior cavity of the body, and of completely protecting them from the effects of gravitation of superimposed parts.

It hence appears that pelvic disease does not result from an unintelligible idiosyncrasy of the affected organs, as popular notion will have it. The real disease, or rather that which demands rectification, is the condition of those vital organs which permits unantagonized gravitation. There is abundant evidence of this, derived from the usual remedial means. All external and internal supports are tacit acknowledgments of the fact. The favorite positions assumed by this class of invalids confirm the statement. The relief they experience from a manual replacement of the womb is additional evidence of the same thing. But neither of these means of relief do anything toward the removal of the cause. Their employment has proved detrimental to recovery, since they practically substitute effect for cause, and thereby favor the repetition of processes and means, from which it is impossible to derive radical effects. Their use, therefore, serves indirectly to perpetuate disease.

But nature is ever ready with her resources.

She will aid us, if we seek and apply her means. Gravitation is just as competent to act in a helpful as in a harmful direction. It is as powerful to remove as to supply obstructions. If we choose, this force will impel from the pelvis with the same energy that it impels toward this region. If we call in its friendly aid, it will yield of its abundant power as an indispensable contribution, cöoperating with every other principle, useful in the desired direction, rendering the aggregate effective and sufficient. Following are descriptions of operations in which gravitation is employed to change the position of the pelvic contents.

5. *MOVEMENT FOR RAISING THE CONTENTS OF THE PELVIS, INVOLVING AID FROM GRAVITATION.*

The patient lies back downward on a horizontal couch, with the hands strongly clasped over the head and pressing on its crown; the feet drawn up so that the heels are in close contact with the trunk, the soles of the feet resting on the couch, the knees and thighs being strongly flexed.

By a moderate effort the patient raises the hips as high as she can, or till the thighs and trunk form a straight line, the shoulders and the feet only resting on the couch; in this position the trunk must for a few moments be sustained. The hips and trunk are now allowed slowly to fall back to the commencing position on the couch. This action may be repeated a half-dozen or more times, a few moments of rest intervening.

If the patient be quite feeble, this movement must be executed with the aid of an assistant. After the position, precisely as described, has been assumed, the assistant's hands are placed under the hips of the patient from either side. Then, by the assistant's own exertions, or by the combined efforts of both, the hips are gently raised but a little higher than by unaided efforts. After a pause, the trunk is allowed to descend slowly to the couch as before.

This movement, whether performed alone or by aid of an assistant, may be practiced several times a day.

In the position assumed by the body at the extreme point to which the hips are raised, it will be observed that the trunk forms an inclined plane, that the hips are many inches higher than the shoulders, and that the pelvis is now above the abdomen, while the latter is higher than the diaphragm. Down the inclined plane thus formed, all the interior organs necessarily tend.

The position of the arms causes distention of the diaphragm and expansion of the space of which the diaphragm is the upper boundary. It has before been seen that the effect of such expansion is to draw toward the increased space the contents below it. But since, in consequence of the position described, these contents inevitably gravitate in the same direction, it follows that muscular action and gravitation now coöperate to the same end. The result is the raising of the contents of the pelvis to a more elevated position.

This movement affords complete relief from the miserable feelings the invalid so often describes as dragging weight in the pelvis, dull aching of the loins, back, or pelvis, with the concomitant general symptoms. It relieves anteversion of the womb, and the frequent desire to pass small quantities of urine, when this is caused by pressure of contiguous parts against the bladder or urethra.

This movement being nearly or entirely passive, according as it is performed with or without an assistant, there is little or no expenditure of the patient's power, and therefore the feeblest invalids are not too weak to receive the benefits derivable from it.

On the other hand, it does not call into active service the sustaining muscles, and therefore but feebly stimulates their nutrition, consequently their sustaining power is less increased by it than by the more active movements. This, however, frequently relieves immediate symptoms, and is an excellent preliminary to, and assistant of, those which produce more decided and permanent effects.

6. *MOVEMENT REQUIRING THE CO-OPERATION OF MUSCULAR POWER WITH GRAVITATION.*

The invalid lies on a horizontal couch, with face downward, the elbows resting firmly on the couch, the arms perpendicular and supporting the upper portion of the trunk, the ankles strongly flexed, the toes, like the elbows, resting firmly on the couch.

By a strong effort all the muscles of the anterior portion, that is, the under side of the body, are caused to contract, the knees are straightened, the hips and whole body raised from the couch, and made to form a horizontal line, touching the couch at no point but the elbows and toes. After sustaining this position for a few moments, or as long as the strength will allow, the body is permitted slowly to recede to its first position, resting on the couch. This operation may be repeated four or five times. The patient will find that the effort required to perform the action now described may be diminished by approximating the points of support, the elbows and the toes.

In the position described, the contents of the abdomen cannot be supported by the pelvis, for they do not gravitate in that direction. These contents now rest upon the anterior walls of the abdomen, and are in a lower horizontal plane than that of the pelvis. It follows that gravitation is shifted to a direction at right angles with that in which it previously acted. In proportion to the lax condition of the abdominal walls will the weight of the abdominal contents tend downward. The effect of this weight is that of traction, or drawing from the pelvis toward the diaphragm.

This effect is caused by position; it is much increased by the effort to raise the central portion of the trunk, necessitated in the act of straightening. In making this endeavor, the walls of the abdomen strongly contract and press their contents forward. As by the position of the arms the diaphragm is expanded, and as the immovable position of the elbows serves to fix it in that condition, it follows that the effort described serves to move forward and, therefore, toward the diaphragm, the whole of the contents of the cavities below it, to fill the space thus provided.

No apparatus being required for its performance, it can be practiced several times a day in one's own room. It is very effective in overcoming retroversion. Indeed this movement affords great and certain relief to women suffering any form of pelvic disorder. This follows from the upward drawing which this action produces on the generative intestine, rectum and bladder.

7. *SIMILAR PROCESS FOR THE SAME PURPOSE, BUT REQUIRING AN ASSISTANT.*

In case of feebleness on the part of the patient, the movement above described may be applied by the aid of an assistant. For this purpose the hands of the assistant (who is in a convenient position by the side of the patient) are placed under the middle portion of the abdomen, and both coöperate in the endeavor to lift the body to the horizontal position. This act may be repeated six or more times, according to the amount of aid furnished by the assistant.

The inability to elevate the body without help arises from the lax, weak condition of the muscles constituting the anterior abdominal walls. The presence of the hand of the assistant at the point exceptionally weak, has a marked effect in increasing the action of the muscles to which they are thus applied. The reason is, that it calls the attention of the patient more energetically to that region, and thus enables her to concentrate her power at the points where it is particularly required. She soon finds that she can exert power in muscles that she had previously been unable to command, and in a short time will from choice perform the operation unaided.

Indeed it is not uncommon, after a few weeks' practice, for the invalid to desire the assistant to supply resistance, instead of affording help. To do this, the assistant places one hand on the back, and the other opposite, under the abdomen. Gentle pressure is now made, adding the resistance of the assistant to that afforded by the weight of the patient's body, just in proportion to her strength, against which the patient raises and straightens her body.

This modification increases the action of the abdominal muscles, and the effect of the movement on the pelvic contents.

8. *MOVEMENT COMBINING GRAVITATION WITH MUSCULAR EFFORT.*

The patient assumes the same position as in No. 6.

Wrapping the folds of the patient's garments closely about her legs, the assistant grasps the feet of the patient and gently lifts the body which is otherwise supported only by the elbows, while the patient carefully maintains the entire body perfectly straight. The limbs may be raised two, three or even more feet from the couch, causing the pelvis to be considerably higher than the chest and abdomen. After remaining a few moments in this position, the body is allowed gradually to return to the couch. This operation may be repeated three or four times, with short intervals of rest.

By this movement the diaphragm is distended to its extreme limit, and fixed by the arms in that position. This increases the amount of space in the upper portion of the abdomen, both upward and laterally. By elevating the inferior portion of the trunk the abdominal muscles are made to act strongly, as in No. 6, pressing forward the abdominal together with the pelvic contents, while the gravitation of the whole contained mass is reversed, and caused to tend toward the diaphragm instead of toward the pelvis. The contents of the cavities of the abdomen and pelvis are forced, by the coöperation of these causes, to assume a more elevated position. The womb is carried forward as well as upward, is disengaged from its position under the promontory of the sacrum, and from its contact with the rectum. The effect of this action is to remove retroversion, with the constipation and other symptoms caused thereby.

Considerable muscular power is required of the patient to sustain the body while being lifted by the feet, as above described. This, however, need be no objection to the employment of the principle of this movement. Its application can be easily modified so as to remove the objection. It is only necessary to grasp the patient at some point nearer the centre of the body, in order to diminish the effort to any extent desired.

In case of thus modifying the application, it is only the muscular action that is diminished, while the expansion of the abdominal space below the diaphragm, together with the effect of gravitation, are quite the same as before. This modification may be employed in case of feebleness, with the result of elevating the womb and its appendages, relieving the pain coincident with the pelvic affections, while it causes no discomfort and little or no fatigue.

9. *MOVEMENT EMPLOYING THE FULL EFFECT OF GRAVITATION.*

The patient lies face downward, the upper portion of the body supported by the elbows, as in No. 6, the lower portion supported by an oblong, narrow and well-padded stool, twelve or fourteen inches in height, placed under the legs, six or eight inches below the flexure of the thighs.

Instead of the stool, the legs of the patient may be supported at the desired elevation by an assistant.

The assistant grasps the legs of the patient, and placing her thighs across the support, employs it as a fulcrum; the body now rests upon the elbows, and the elevated support. The assistant presses the legs downward, which act, in consequence of the position of the fulcrum, causes her hips to rise, so elevating the body as to cause it to make the line of its inclination very steep; the legs are immediately raised, causing a return to the former position. This action of alternately depressing and raising is repeated six or eight times, after which the patient resumes her position on the couch.

This action is nearly passive, tasking the muscles of the abdomen and pelvis to only a moderate degree. The inclination assumed by the trunk being great, more effect is secured from gravitation than is derivable from other movements. The muscular action which is excited cooperates with this effect of gravitation, and the contents of the cavities of the body are urged toward the diaphragm to an extreme degree.

The motion of alternate raising and depressing the thighs calls into action certain muscles whose function is to flex and to twist the legs, and whose action in the upright position, as in walking, gives rise to local discomfort and even pain. The effect of the action of these muscles in the position described is to relieve pain. Their action aids the effect of position in transferring the visceral organs to a more elevated plane.

This movement is also particularly useful to disengage the fundus of the retroverted womb from its position, when it has been long fixed under the promontory of the sacrum and has mechanically pressed upon the rectum, preventing the action of the bowels. It serves the purpose more efficiently in some cases than others of its class, in removing the impacted condition of the pelvic contents, and all their severe and otherwise unmanageable consequences affecting the local as well as the general health.

The power of this movement to restore the displaced uterus is very great. A good deal of preliminary treatment is usually necessary in order to bring the muscles into a condition to retain, permanently, the restored position. After due preparation, I have known the uterus which had long lain nearly horizontal in the anterio-posterior diameter of the pelvis, to be quite restored in a few days through the employment of this, aided by similar movements. Even the severest cases of retroversion become perfectly tractable under these means.

10. *MOVEMENT EMPLOYING BOTH MUSCULAR ACTION AND GRAVITATION, FACILITATED AND GRADUATED BY APPARATUS.*

Description of Apparatus.—A plain narrow couch, having an upholstered top, is provided. To this is attached a quadrilateral frame of its exact width, resting evenly with its top. This frame is caused to rise from the couch by means of its connection through pivots at its central portion, with a lever beneath, which is acted on by the foot of the assistant. Broad and well upholstered pads are laid across the frames at whatever point it is desired the body of the patient should be sustained.

The patient lies face downward upon the couch thus arranged, so that one of the pads shall be under her chest, while the arms rest upon the frame, and the other pad is under the legs; the whole resting upon the couch.

The assistant, placing her foot upon the lever and steadying the frame with her hand, depresses the lever, and raises the frame upon which the patient is sustained by the transverse pads. The body is thus raised several inches above the couch, and touches nothing but the pads on which it rests. It is essential that the patient, at the same time, maintains her form in a perfectly straight line, not allowing the body to fall through the interspace between the pads; this is done by the action of the muscles of the abdomen and the inferior portion of the body. It is necessary that the muscular action, and the bodily sustentation which is its consequence, should be uninterrupted during the time the body is raised from the couch.

While thus raised, the weight of the body is supported by the two pivots of the frame near its centre, and it is consequently very nearly balanced. The assistant, who steadies the frame and the body it supports with one hand, can easily cause one extremity to rise above the other at will, or either extremity to become higher in alternation. If this action be practiced, the time the patient can easily sustain her position can be considerably prolonged, since the change in the hydrostatic relations of the circulation produces a restful effect.

After thus sustaining the patient for a few moments, the pressure of the foot upon the lever may gradually relax, and the body will slowly fall to its original position on the couch. This operation may be repeated four or five times.

This apparatus is equally appropriate for those who have full strength and those who have none, since the degree of effect its use produces is entirely controlled by the adjustment of its sustaining pads. These may be so placed that the weight of the body is equally divided upon them. In this case the body is in a state of perfect equipoise, and there is no muscular strain or action induced.

If, however, these pads be placed a little farther apart, more weight comes between them than is balanced by the extremities, and an effort is instinctively made by the abdominal muscles to sustain the body and prevent it from sinking between the supports; this effort should be augmented by the will. The necessity for effort to sustain the body, and for action of the muscles that perform this duty, increases in exact proportion to the distance asunder the pads are removed.

When the patient is raised on this apparatus in the manner above described, the following effects are produced. The space at the upper region of the abdomen is increased by the position of the arms. The abdomen gravitates at right angles to its previous direction, which relieves the pelvis of all superimposed weight. The abdominal muscles are caused so to act as to impel their contents forward, toward the diaphragm. At the will of the operator the forward end of the frame is depressed, and, being pivoted in the middle, the opposite end is elevated. This causes the pelvis to be the highest, and of course the visceral organs to gravitate from the pelvis, drawing its contents forward and upward.

It will be observed that the use of this apparatus combines several forces, and causes them to coöperate in one direction, producing the effect of removing from the pelvis the chief causes of its sufferings.

This apparatus has a remarkable adaptation to all classes of cases, even if the abdominal muscles be too weak to contract in this position; still, being unsupported between the pads, the advantages derivable from gravitation are secured to the pelvis, so that the favorable effects of the operation are soon felt, and the more decided and permanent ones of muscular action and development directly follow.

Similar effects may be secured, without apparatus or assistant, in the following manner:

Two stools or chairs are placed so far asunder that the patient in lying face downward across them will be supported by the chest resting upon one, and the legs upon the other. While thus lying, the abdomen is unsupported, and consequently gravitates toward the ground, causing retraction of the generative intestine. In this position, the patient must endeavor to maintain her body in a straight line, in opposition to the force of gravity acting on its central portion.

She can also graduate the force of the movement by changing the relative position of her two supports. If able to sustain more weight, she can place the supports farther asunder; if less, she can approximate them; and in this way she can with advantage test her own strength and secure the rectification of the position of internal organs, and the development of those muscles which control these relations. A woman who suspects in herself a tendency to disease of the pelvis, is by means of this process easily able to avert it—strengthening the parts on whose weakness the inroad of disease depends, before the more serious question of cure can arise.

XIII.

MEANS FOR INCREASING THE POWER AND ACTION OF THE MUSCLES OF THE ABDOMEN.

THE aims of all treatment designed for the prevention and cure of diseases pertaining to the pelvis are but imperfectly fulfilled by the restoration of the correct position of the organs or by the apparent removal of the diseased state. The ordinary treatment fails of achieving the desired results, because of its restricted purposes. Instruments may hold the uterus in place, and active depletion may reduce engorgement, but it does not follow that these remedies effect restoration. Unless these and other beneficial effects are continuous, the improved condition of the patient cannot be maintained.

It has been shown that engorgement of the pelvic organs and its results do not occur as a consequence of the need of depletion, but from deficient power to carry forward the circulation at this particular part of its course. So also it is not the need of the supporting instrument which causes deviation of the womb, but the need of supporting muscular power and action.

It hence appears that the true preventive as well as the rational remedial measures must consist in the development of the muscular powers, which affords the required support, and which also assures the profound reciprocal action of respiration. The following are some of the processes best calculated to effect this purpose:

11. *MOVEMENT REQUIRING ACTION OF THE ABDOMINAL WALLS AT EACH SIDE.*

The patient sits upon a stool, one hand placed firmly upon her hips, fingers forward, the arm of the other side stretched directly upward parallel with the trunk, the knees wide apart, feet resting on the floor, but held immovably in place by appropriate straps, or by being placed under some weighty article of furniture, convenient for restraining them.

The trunk is allowed slowly to fall diagonally backward and sidewise, in the direction of the side having the hand upon the hip, to a distance proportioned to the ability to rise. This distance may be progressively greater, according to the increase of power, and will finally reach a point below the horizontal. The trunk slowly resumes its first or perpendicular position. This act may be repeated three or four times, after which the position of the arms may be exchanged, and the action repeated in the new position, the trunk falling in the opposite diagonal direction.

This movement calls into energetic use the muscles of each lateral half of the abdomen and of the chest. The acting side of the chest becomes elevated, which causes an increase of space at that side of the abdomen both upward and laterally, and the coincident contraction of the abdominal walls of the same side compels the contents of the cavity to a more elevated position. The nutrition and power of the abdominal muscles being thus increased, they gradually participate more and more in the respiratory motions. This both prevents the undue effect of gravitation and removes these effects when existing.

If there be sufficient strength, this movement may be performed with a light weight grasped by the upstretched hand. The action of the muscles of the chest and abdomen is increased in proportion to the amount of weight.

12. *THE SAME AIDED BY AN ASSISTANT.*

The patient is in the same position as described in No. 11. An assistant grasps the upstretched arm near the wrist with one hand, while the other supports the opposite shoulder of the patient. The trunk executes the same apparent action as in No. 11. But the assistant adjusts the resistance to the acting muscles, instead of this being left to the weight of the body. In the beginning of the motion, the patient offers slight resistance, which the assistant overcomes by pressing the trunk backward and sidewise. When the point is reached where the resistance is too great for the falling body to bear, a portion of its weight is sustained by the assistant, who also controls the time in which the operation is performed. In returning to the erect position, the assistant first aids in raising the trunk, which aid is gradually diminished as the trunk approaches the upright position, till near its end when resistance is offered. The resistance may be increased with the increasing strength of the patient.

It will be found that the resistance supplied by an assistant produces an effect on the patient quite different and very superior to that of an inanimate weight. The former is not only adjusted with minute exactness to the varying power of the patient's muscles throughout the whole extent of their action, but it more thoroughly and vigorously than the latter stimulates this action, and at the same time is followed by less fatigue. The cause is probably referable to some not yet understood relation between the nervous systems of the two coöperating parties, the explanation of which we must be content to forego. The effect of this movement has already been sufficiently explained.

13. *MOVEMENT CALLING INTO ACTION ALL THE ANTERIOR MUSCLES OF THE ABDOMEN.*

The patient sits upright, with back unsupported, the feet firmly fixed upon the floor, the hands clasped and resting on the crown of the head. The trunk is allowed to fall directly backward, slowly, as far as the strength is able to support the weight in this position, it then slowly rises till its first or perpendicular position is regained. This action may be repeated four or five times, and may be varied by putting the arms in a perpendicular position, which, by affording more leverage for their weight, causes more resistance and compels more action of the muscles of the abdomen. This form of the movement can be taken only by those who are comparatively strong, or when they have by practice acquired much strength. A weaker class of invalids may place their hands upon their hips, and thus diminish the resistance and action of the muscles. Or what is better, an assistant may aid in the performance of the operation, by placing her hands on the shoulders of the patient, and while the movement is in progress, may afford resistance at points where it is needed, and aid in sustaining the weight when the task is too severe for the muscles.

The effect is quite similar to that of the two last described, but more than double the amount of muscle is engaged, which renders the operation more severe and fatiguing. For this reason it need be repeated but two or three times, especially until the strength has improved. The attention and the conditions for nutritive action are powerfully directed to the abdominal muscles, while the diaphragm is distended and elevated.

TWISTING THE TRUNK.

The importance of the class of motions and exercises which cause the body to become slightly twisted, and the general principles of such actions, have been explained on page 69, to which the reader is referred. Following is a description of a few movements of this class, with a further description of their effects.

14. *MOVEMENT DEVELOPING THE OBLIQUE AND TRANSVERSE MUSCLES OF THE ABDOMEN.*

The position the same as in No. 13. The trunk may be perpendicular, or it may recline a little, according to the strength; the latter position requiring much more power to execute the movement than the former.

An assistant grasps the patient's arms near the elbows, and while the patient slowly *twists* her trunk to the right, the assistant offers gentle resistance. The patient next twists her trunk in the opposite direction, to the left, again overcoming the resistance offered by the assistant. The extent of the twisting action is limited only by the ability of the parts to move in either direction. This action may be repeated three or four times each way.

The abdominal muscles, chiefly those which lie in the transverse and in the diagonal direction, are those to which the action of this movement is principally confined. The position of the arms causes the chest and diaphragm to be expanded and rigidly fixed, which, as has been shown, secures the greatest space in the upper abdominal or epigastric region. Since the length of the trunk is maintained by the spine under all circumstances, it follows that a twisting motion, whether passive or active, causes strong compression of the abdomen. The voluntary contraction of the muscles of the abdomen, produced by the twisting effort, adds greatly to this effect. These causes coöperate in contracting the lower portion of the abdomen and in pressing upon its contents; and now by the expanded condition of the diaphragm, and consequent increased space immediately beneath it, the abdominal contents are both invited and forced in an upward direction, counteracting their tendency to press upon the pelvic contents.

15. *THE SAME WITHOUT ASSISTANCE.*

Position of patient the same as in No. 14, but the assistant is dispensed with.

The trunk is turned or twisted to each side alternately by the patient's voluntary efforts.

The rate of motion may vary from that of extreme slowness to that of great rapidity. It may be repeated twenty or more times, care being taken during the operation to maintain the same axis of motion, and to have the direction of motion at right angles with its axis, and to avoid any tendency to rotary motion.

The amount of power required for this exercise depends on the degree of deviation of the trunk from the perpendicular, and should be proportioned to the ability of the patient.

The effect is similar to that described under No. 14, except that it is productive of more fatigue.

If, however, the movement be accelerated, other distinct and often very desirable effects are secured. The circulation becomes excited, much centrifugal effect is produced, respiration is increased, and there is a great increase of bodily heat and perspiration. These effects are those of stimulation.

16. *TWISTING MOVEMENT OF THE TRUNK.*

The patient lies on a horizontal couch, the hands clasped over the head, and pressing strongly upon its crown, the feet drawn up in close contact with the body, and resting firmly on the couch.

An assistant presses upon the shoulders of the patient, so as to maintain them in close contact with the couch, while another assistant grasps both knees, and presses them slowly to one side, against the resistance of the patient, till the knees come in contact with the couch. The patient continuing her efforts, causes the knees and legs to move in the opposite direction, opposing the resistance of the assistant, which is continued till the knees and legs reach the couch at the opposite side. The direction of the motion is again changed, bringing the corresponding muscles of the opposite side into action, the assistant continuing to resist so as to excite the more effective endeavors of the patient. This may be repeated four or five times slowly.

This movement may be taken without the aid of an assistant, but produces much less effect.

This motion twists the trunk, and therefore brings into strong action the transverse and oblique muscles of the abdomen, and produces effects similar to those described in No. 14. It may be preferred in case it be desirable to avoid the upright position, as when there is great weakness.

Other modifications of the twisting action may be employed by putting the body in other positions, as for example, standing with the hands placed on the hips, or grasping some fixed object above, or in the lying, face downward, position, &c. These, in general, require the aid of an assistant.

17. *MOVEMENT FOR ELEVATING THE CONTENTS OF THE ABDOMEN AND PELVIS, AND TO STRENGTHEN THE SUSTAINING PARTS.*

The patient kneels on a couch or cushioned seat, near its edge, with trunk erect, arms extended forward and parallel, and hands resting on the shoulders of an assistant, who stands immediately in front of and facing her. The patient is steadied by the hands of the assistant being placed under and supporting her shoulders. It is better to have the feet of the patient held firmly in position.

The assistant slowly retreats a step, perhaps two, drawing the upper part of the patient's body forward and causing it to incline strongly in that direction, the assistant stooping in proportion to the distance of the retreat, so as to accommodate the elevation of the shoulders which support the patient, to her height, which is diminished as the upper portion of her body advances. While thus falling forward, the patient must be particularly careful to maintain the body quite straight, avoiding all bending at the hips. The distance the upper part of the body is caused to advance will depend on the strength of the patient. After due practice, the advance may be continued until the horizontal position of the body is attained. After reaching the point desired, the trunk is returned to its commencing or perpendicular position. This action may be repeated three or four times.

With every inch of advance in this operation, the ribs are drawn apart and raised, the diaphragm distended, and the superior abdominal space increased, till at the terminal position these ends are attained in an extreme degree. This effect is an inevitable consequence of the relation of the chest muscles to the arms. At the same time, the weight of the body is so thrown forward of its usual support that the abdominal muscles are compelled to coöperate in sustaining it, and prevent the trunk from bending unduly forward. This produces upward pressure upon the abdominal contents at the same instant that the action of the muscles of the chest is providing space in the upper portion of the cavity. The result is a very strong elevating effect secured for the contents of the abdomen. This upward action extends demonstrably to the contents of the pelvis, relieving them of congestion, and other consequences of superincumbent weight.

18. *MOVEMENT COMBINING THE ACTION OF CHEST AND DIAPHRAGM, WITH TWISTING OF THE TRUNK.*

Position as in No. 17. The action differs from that movement in this: as the upper portion of the body is drawn forward, it is directed to one side of the assistant, and thus the trunk is rotated on its axis, so that the face of the patient will present toward the assistant instead of directly forward, causing the trunk to become slightly twisted, while the legs remain as before. The patient is returned to commencing position, as in the last.

This action combines in a high degree all the effects described in No. 11 and No. 17. The patient requires considerable practice in the two movements referred to, before she can readily coöperate with the assistant. After this power is acquired, the movement will be found to secure the most gratifying effects in diseases of the pelvic contents.

XIV.

KNEADING THE ABDOMEN. COMBINATION OF KNEADING WITH MUSCULAR ACTION AND GRAVITATION.

THE feasibility and importance of increasing the development as well as the power of the muscles by judicious exercise is too obvious and generally accepted to need further enforcement. But it remains to be shown that such exercise may be superinduced by other than the usual means, for the benefit of a large class of invalids.

Muscular action is ordinarly induced by the will. When we speak of exercise, we usually mean those actions and motions of the muscular system that originate in and are controlled by our own volition. But action originating outside the body may be produced in the muscles, and made to reach every fibre and cell of the muscular system without the least effort of will on the patient's part, and consequently without the least expenditure of force. This action may be communicated to the system by the hand of an operator, or through the medium of mechanism designed for and adapted to this purpose. In the former case, the patient exercises her body, the consequent fatigue oftentimes doing more harm than the exercise does good; in the latter case, her body is exercised, and without the least fatigue, while the beneficial motion is communicated directly to those parts of the system which most need invigoration.

This method of exercise is so little understood, and the effects of action communicated to the system from without are so unfamiliar even to medical practitioners generally, that it may be well to explain both its principles and effects before giving specific directions.

In ordinary exercise, the brain and nerves, which are chiefly concerned in all manifestations of will-power, are first called into action, and the motion is thence extended to the muscles. The brain and nerves are consequently exercised quite as much, if not more, than the muscles; and it follows that the nutritive results of action are proportionally divided between the muscular and nervous elements, and they are thus prepared for succeeding actions.

But in case the exercise is applied by some

person or instrument, or agency outside the system, the result is changed. The brain and nerves, the instruments of the will, are spared participation in the work; the nutritive result will hence be chiefly dispensed to the muscles, which are now the only acting parts. It follows that by supplying action in this way, the very important advantage may be gained of giving increased nutrition and consequent strength to the muscles, while the nerves remain quiescent.

In case of great muscular weakness, the effects of exertion, or voluntary action, are quite the reverse of what they are in health. For in proportion to the incapacity of the muscles is the demand on the nervous resources increased. Want of strength, in other words, must be compensated for by increased efforts. What the muscles lack the nervous system is taxed to supply. And since nutrition follows the demand produced by action, it is plain that the disparity between these channels of force is rendered greater. Hence, if those suffering from weakness of muscles are subjected to strong voluntary efforts, the muscles become weaker rather than stronger, while the preponderance of nervous power and activity increases.

That such are the actual results of the efforts of feeble women, is amply confirmed by experience. Women with disordered pelvic organs are indisposed to action, they are admonished by bitter experience to forbear exercise, and there is insufficient power for its execution. Injury to the pelvic organs is often asserted as its effect, but the local consequences are quite insignificant compared to the mal-distributions of force, which are the concomitant effects. The increased feebleness of muscular power and the nervous irritability which succeed disproportioned efforts are confirmations of these statements.

Such are the common and well-known experiences of feeble women. They are just the opposite of what is desired. The objects sought are more muscular and less nerve nutrition and action. These are attainable only by such action as shall suspend the will-power and the nerve-excitation, while the nutritive action of the muscles is promoted. Hence it is clear that for therapeutical ends, *the predominant action must be passive*; and it must be communicated to the system by some person or agency without making the least draft upon the enfeebled resources of the invalid.

The process for securing the effects above described for the abdomen, including both the muscular walls and the visceral organs, is called *kneading*. Some form of manipulating, as well described by this as by any other term, has always been practiced among all primitive people the world over, having its justification wholly in experience. The great value of the process for chronic invalids is proved by the effects it produces wherever patience and perseverance have been exercised in its application.

The use of the kneading process is evident from the analogy afforded by animals. All inferior creatures subject the abdominal walls and contents to vigorous action at every step of their locomotion. These walls are thereby healthfully tasked, and their contents beneficially disturbed. The good effect of this motion is much increased by increase of pace.

In the human species, the want of this motion is compensated by another power which is nearly denied the animal; viz., the power of bending, and especially that of twisting, the body in the upright position. All such motions not only serve to strengthen the abdominal walls and contents, and to stimulate their functions, but produce a like effect on the contents of the pelvis. These principles were fully explained on page 69.

The process of kneading, then, simply supplies the motions that have been long neglected. The neglect of these motions is inevitably followed by loss of capacity for exercise, and involves the necessity of some substitute in order to maintain the functional processes of the system. Hence the resort of modern civilized people to remedies of quite another sort, losing sight of the virtues of the old, well-tried and proved process of kneading. The advantages of this application of force have been vainly sought among the usual resources of the medical art. For, leaving out of sight the temporary emergencies which may be well administered to by appropriate medicines, it is difficult to conceive the use or relevancy of internal medication for the main indication,—weakness of muscle.

Permanent increase of muscular power can be secured only in one way, by the action of the part requiring these effects. No other remedy has yet achieved any reputation as a substitute for such action. And, in spite of the abundant prescribings with which the feeble woman is overwhelmed, it is still futile to expect to increase the capacity and power of the instruments of force in her system in any other way. Nature cannot be successfully defeated of her purposes. The coverings of the abdomen are muscular, and these muscles imperatively call for nutritive support. The contained parts are also muscular, and notwithstanding their function of conveying and digesting nutritive materials, they are strengthened by exterior excitation. In civilized life the necessities imposed on the muscles are diminished. With females these demands are very few, and much inferior to the physiological needs. In many cases the voluntary call for such action is quite absent. Decline of power is therefore inevitable. Those who are losing power are practically cut off from the conditions for its reparation; and if they have approached helplessness, they are generally doomed to a long period of invalidism, which the direct and appropriate remedy might speedily remove.

The process of kneading the abdomen quite meets the needs of the condition pointed out. Being entirely passive, it produces no fatigue. It directs nutrition to the parts subjected to the process, and is followed by rapid increase of muscular power of the internal organs as well as their coverings. The abdomen even acquires a good degree of solidity and hardness to the touch. The process acts as a revulsive to the spine, relieving its congestion. It always proves restful in fatigue. The extremities and skin become warm, and filled with blood under its influence, and a strong disposition to sleep steals over the patient, even under the operation. These effects become directly apparent after a few applications, and afford a strong presumption that this method of treatment will lead to the most important results, if not to a permanent cure.

We may therefore confidently depend on kneading the abdomen to afford the desired aid in restoring the contractile power, whose loss has been regarded throughout this work as most influential among the causes of disease of the pelvic region.

For constipation, indigestion, and the numerous symptoms connected therewith, it is probable that manipulating the abdomen will prove beneficial, even though the process be indifferently applied. But if there be pelvic disease, much care is necessary to render the operation beneficial. The effect will depend entirely on the METHOD of its administration. Injurious effects may readily be produced by careless methods of applying the process. The negative results or the positive injury that has followed misapplication of kneading has doubtless destroyed the confidence of many who have experimented with it. The difficulty arises from want of definite aim, the lack of study of the purposes to be attained, and the want of skill that can be obtained only by experience.

What desirable object, for example, is attained by roughly handling the abdomen, and applying irregular and uncontrolled pressure to that part of the body while lying upon the back? The force expended in such operations is directed downward, and consequently toward the pelvis, and it inevitably pushes the abdominal contents down upon those of the pelvis. This is exactly the reverse of the needs of the case, and opposed to all healthful results. The process thus applied can hardly fail to aggravate the previously existing diseased condition. Only when the patient has considerable muscular strength are these prejudicial effects obviated.

It hence appears that if beneficent effects are to be derived from the power of kneading, this process must be applied on some other principle than that described. Indeed it would seem necessary to quite reverse the process and cause the patient to lie face downward, and the kneading motion and pressure to be applied in the upward and forward direction.

By applying the process of kneading in this position and manner, not only is the liability to negative and injurious effects entirely avoided, but all those beneficial effects for which the process is naturally invoked are easily and perfectly attained.

The reader will clearly understand the advantages of this position by reference to Chaps. V. and XII. Not only is the weight of the abdomen in this position removed from the pelvis, but this weight actually serves as a tractile force upon the pelvic contents, drawing them upward and forward in the direction of the diaphragm. The kneading process must necessarily be applied from beneath. We are now prepared to examine in detail the effects attainable by the process as thus applied.

18. *KNEADING THE ABDOMEN WITHOUT APPARATUS.*

The patient lies face downward, the breast supported by a chair or stool, and the legs by another, the supports being placed from twelve to twenty inches asunder.

An assistant standing by the side of and bending over the patient, easily reaches the abdomen. With the hands firmly clenched, an upward and inward motion may be applied alternately to both sides of the unsupported abdomen.

Another Method. The patient lying in the position last described, the assistant assumes by her side the half-kneeling position, (one knee on the floor and the other in contact with the patient's body, the foot resting on the floor,) and using the horizontal thigh as a fulcrum, the arm of the assistant is used as a lever, and reaching the abdomen with a rigidly clenched hand, gives it the successive impulses which constitute kneading. The other hand of the assistant is employed to sustain and steady the patient.

Every impulse thus given upward is immediately followed by an equal motion downward, produced by gravitation. The upward motion cannot press upon the pelvis, though it may lift the whole body. It merely antagonizes the gravitation of the parts upon which it impinges. The downward motion draws toward the line of its axis all connected parts. Such parts as are mobile, acquire motion in that direction. The germinal intestine, with the rectum and bladder, are by this motion moved upward, or rather in the direction that would be upward in the standing posture, but which is downward in the position now occupied.

It will hence be seen that if the kneading be applied in the forward lying position, two forces are involved in the process. One is the impinging force of the kneading agent, which in any other position constitutes the whole process. The other is the force of gravity, rendered operative by the upward lifting of the kneading power.

This is repeated as often as is the kneading action. The amount of gravitation brought into operation is exactly equal to the impinging force. A portion of this force acts *toward* the central portion of the abdomen, and consequently *from* the pelvis, and thus removes pressure upon its contents.

The amount of force acting upon the mobile parts of the cavity of the abdomen is doubled by this mode of applying the kneading process, and the effect, including the traction upon the pelvic contents, is, by the position, still further increased.

There is, however, a serious difficulty to be overcome in the application of kneading on the principle now explained. This is the extreme labor and fatigue to which the operator is subjected. The position and the direction in which the force is applied involve great expenditure of power, and it is practically found that fatigue compels discontinuance of the operation before the due effect is secured.

This difficulty, nevertheless, proved more seeming than real. It served a useful purpose, that of stimulating efforts to overcome it, which finally became successful, in the production of various kneading instruments. Some of these instruments are worked by an assistant, some are driven by power derived from other sources. Those worked by an assistant require but a small amount of power; if worked by other means, the advantage is had of greater regularity and constancy of motion. In either case, the action of the instrument is under the entire control of the one for whom it is used; on this account the action can never be otherwise than agreeable to the patient, since she can at any moment adjust its degree to suit her feelings and wishes; she can cause it to perform more delicately, or cease entirely.

There are modifications of these instruments in which gravitation is employed to aid the working force. Thus this agency, through the intervention of mechanical adaptations, is rendered as servicable for curative purposes as it had before been instrumental in producing injury.

19. *APPARATUS FOR KNEADING, TO BE WORKED BY OTHER THAN MUSCULAR POWER.*

The apparatus required to apply this process resembles a couch, upon which the invalid reclines face downwards. The top is well upholstered, admits of being adjusted to any elevation, and has a wide opening through which the motion derived from the instrument may reach the body. By means of appropriate connections, the ends of a lever, which is pivoted in its middle portion, together with the kneading-heads they bear, are made to travel in a perpendicular circle by the requisite connections with steam power. These heads impinge against the abdomen, during the upward and forward portion of the circular motion they describe.

While the kneading-heads press against the abdomen, they at the same time move three or four inches upward and forward—that is, toward the diaphragm. This motion necessarily carries with it the portion of the abdomen which it engages by pressure at each revolution. The two heads act alternately upon the sides of the body. The rate of motion should be about fifty or sixty per minute. More rapid motion does the work less effectually: even slower rates are often desirable.

This process combines the force of gravitation with that of mechanism, both contributing to the same result. For in the position described, the unsupported weight of the abdomen draws upward and forward from the pelvis, while the action communicated from the kneading-heads to the same parts moves the visceral organs in the same direction. The soft, yielding nature of the abdomen and convoluted form and gliding quality of the organs, render this result of the process easy and certain.

This apparatus is so modified as to be operated by the foot of an assistant.

Its external appearance is that of a common stool with a broad opening through its top. This is placed between two chairs, and across these the patient lies, precisely as in the last process. Beneath this stool the kneading portion of the apparatus is fixed and operated by the foot of the assistant placed upon one end of the pivoted lever, while the other end is balanced by a weight. The slightest pressure of the foot produces the desired motion of the kneading-heads, which is very similar to that of the last-described apparatus. By means of this arrangement whatever motion is imparted to the lever by the foot is communicated through the connections described, to the abdomen.

Of other methods of kneading for the purpose of securing upward traction from the pelvis, one more is selected for description in this place.

20. *KNEADING WITH ROLLERS.*

A couch like that described in No. 19 constitutes the foundation of the apparatus.

Immediately under the opening is a transverse shaft, which may be revolved by a crank, or by means of power derived from any adequate source. Affixed to this shaft are short arms having axes, which bear broad rollers of small diameter.

At each revolution of the shaft, these rollers are passed through the opening at the top of the couch, and into contact with the body lying upon it. These rollers impinge alternately upon the abdomen, with an upward and forward motion, at every revolution of the shaft. By means of adjusting the arms, the extent of the arc of the circle in which these rollers act can be controlled according to convenience.

The transfer of the contents of the cavities of the trunk upward is very distinctly felt during this process. The effect is similar to that described in No. 19.

In estimating the effects of kneading the abdomen on the principles now explained, time is an important element. In severe cases of retroversion or even of prolapsus, a single operation of this kind may *seem* to have no efficacy whatever, as indeed it may not, so far as immediate symptoms are concerned. But in some degree the effect desired has really been secured, to which daily additions may be made in increasing ratio, as the basis for improvement is gradually made broader. The patient must consider that at each operation these several elements of reparation have been aided:

1. The muscles of the abdominal walls have had their nutrition increased and their substance hardened by the action they have received.

2. Visceral congestion has been removed by

providing a use for the surplus contents of the pelvic vessels.

3. A degree of counter-irritation, producing distinct revulsive effects, has been established.

4. More space has been provided at the epigastric region, toward which the hypogastric contents have distinctly and demonstrably moved.

5. The tendency of the womb to fall or to bend back upon the rectum has diminished from the first application of the process. When the womb is moved to its place by the sound, it is forced against the pressure of the digestive organs, and is by them immediately pushed back to its abnormal and distressful position on the removal of the sound. Not so now. The womb rises of itself to its natural position as space is provided for it by the elevating of the digestive organs. This elevation is gradually but surely secured by the processes described, and the overlying mass ceases to act as the cause of disease.

The patient receiving this treatment will not, of course, expect the immediate removal of her sufferings. She will not experience effects similar to those of the sedative to which she may be accustomed; nor will the symptoms, during the intervals of treatment, reappear with full vigor, as they do after the influence of a quieting drug has passed away. Even if the symptoms peculiar to her case should at first be a little aggravated, they should not be regarded seriously. The disturbance of the pelvic contents by the processes will often arouse new but transient sensations, indicative of a resumption of power. But the characteristic symptoms of her disease will gradually and quite certainly disappear, especially if the effects of kneading be well supported by the judicious use of operations heretofore described. The patient should feel a confidence in these *principles*, and carry out a firm determination to rely upon them, and her ultimate triumph over pelvic hyperæmia and its numerous outgrowths will be complete and unequivocal. She will be disappointed in finding the processes and applications far easier and more agreeable than her imagination had depicted, and will, in consequence, be inclined to overdo during the first few days of her treatment. She is cautioned against this.

The importance of the kneading process for the purposes I have now indicated has been most unaccountably overlooked by the medical profession. It does not hesitate to supply mechanical aids for weakness and deformities of the extremities. It recommends and devises instruments, and counsels the employment of manipulations, frictions, special exercises, and whatever will contribute to physiological action for the cure of these ailments.

The affections of the contents of the female pelvis I have shown to consist of both weakness and deformity—weakness of dominant parts and deformity accompanying the pathological condition of the organs, and that the indications of treatment are exceedingly clear and distinct. I have also shown the peculiar amenability of the pelvic region to treatment, and that the facility with which affections of this region yield to the treatment which I have shown to be appropriate is exceptional in the practice of the healing art. It will next be shown that the success attainable through any other channel is the consequence of the practical application of these principles.

The principles involved in the treatment of disorders and diseases of the contents of the pelvis, as developed in the foregoing chapters, embrace several distinct purposes, which may be summarized as follows:

First. An improved distribution of the circulation. Pelvic, like all other congestion, is powerfully antagonized by well-directed endeavors to circulate the blood more freely in the extremities and skin. Treatment which neglects this purpose, however appropriate it otherwise may be, can have but feeble influence in removing disease whose essence is congestion of a central region or organ.

Second. Expansion of the diaphragm and of the space immediately beneath it, so as to produce room for the visceral contents at a greater elevation in the cavity of the trunk. This induces expansion of the chest and increase of the degree of the reciprocating motions of respiration, extending these motions to the abdomen and pelvis.

Third. Contraction of the lower portion of the abdominal walls, and the increase of the power of the muscles which constitute the walls. The action of the muscles sustains the abdominal contents, and prevents their pressure upon those of the pelvis.

Fourth. The employment of gravitation, the

intermediate cause of pelvic affections, as an active and efficient agent of restoration.

Fifth. The employment of mechanical adaptations, to be operated by other than human power, to exercise and harden the defective muscles of the very weakly and helpless, and to transfer the contents of the abdomen and pelvis to a higher place in the cavity of the trunk.

XV.

DEMONSTRATION OF THE EFFECTS OF PROCESSES.

THE therapeutic processes herein developed have their sole basis in anatomy and physiology —in the very mechanism and uses of the body. They set in action a self-regenerating machine. They do what health ordinarily does to insure its own continuance. This is in strong contrast with methods which rely on the dubious relation existing between vitality and a multitude of substances exerting chemical force—a relation always obscure, and affording good ground for differing and conflicting opinions.

The ease and directness with which the truth of these statements of principles and effects of processes can be demonstrated should silence all question as to their correctness and feasibility —the curative effects asserted are readily confirmed. No faith is demanded. There are no mysterious and unintelligible relations of things involved. The invalid's own capacities are exercised and judgment appealed to. Ample directions are given for verification by direct personal experiment. Certain specific effects are practically connected with their causes. As a lover of truth, I shall be heartily thankful for every honest application of these tests that shall expose the incorrectness, if there be any, of the principles stated or the inferences drawn.

Rightly understood, the therapeutic principles and means here advocated cannot justly be regarded as inimical to other current methods. All medical practice is founded on differences, and therefore choice, of remedies. Experience develops progress in a science as in an individual. The good is displaced by the better; but the latter depends on the former, and is not opposed to it.

As to statements of the experience of invalids in the use of remedies, there has always been much unwitting deception practiced. Such statements should in general be taken with exceeding caution. This is because there are two principles engaged in the curative process, vitality and the remedial agency, and it is well nigh impossible to determine properly their respective influences. For this reason the greatest credit is sometimes given where there is least merit.

The therapeutic principles and measures proposed are singularly free from this difficulty. But one of the above-mentioned factors is brought into use, and whatever credit there may be, must be due to it. This one is nature asserting its powers assisted by physiological and mechanical conditions, and the remedial element of doubtful influence is eliminated.

The idea underlying the principles discussed in this work had its beginning in the following manner:

Many years ago I was consulted by a gentleman, a prominent member of the Bench, occupying a high social position, for professional aid. He had been treated for chronic diarrhœa. Its peculiarities, however, engaged my interest. The motions were frequent, but ineffectual, accompanied by much straining, which always caused a portion of the rectum to protrude beyond the sphincter. This necessitated its manual replacement after every attempted evacuation.

His *real* disease proved to be *prolapsus of the bowels.* The diarrhœa was but a *symptom,* and was solely due to an extension upward of the irritation derived from the often protruding rectum, and thus affecting, probably, a considerable tract of the intestinal membrane, but did not exist as an idiopathic affection.

The case was chronic; it had not improved under eminent skill; books of surgery, and consultation with a well-known surgeon, afforded but dubious prospects of satisfactory advantage from medical treatment.

This case proved, however, to afford one of those occasions in which the stimulus of extraordinary need evokes corresponding benefits, where the aid sought is suddenly and unexpectedly secured.

While applying some obviously needed palliative, the patient for this purpose assuming the forward lying position, the idea presented itself which forms the fundamental one of the present treatise. I carefully placed him in the position described on page 174. I then desired him to make the peculiar effort there described, at the same time encouraging the endeavor and assisting the action of the muscles, as before directed. I had the supreme satisfaction of actually *seeing* the effect. The protruding, swollen, and very tender part *instantly slipped in, and wholly disappeared.*

This and other similar experiments were pregnant with suggestions destined to culminate in important results. Some of them may be stated as follows:

The power required to elevate the intestine can easily be applied from above.

The power is more effective if applied from above, because the whole alimentary tube is thus raised, for when the visceral mass is moved upward the terminal extremity must follow, while if the moving power be applied below but a minute portion is acted upon.

The upward movement described reveals the existence of sustaining elements. Any operation applied from beneath recognizes no such element.

Effects thus attained would pass into a permanent condition, by increasing the power of the sustaining elements.

These sustaining elements consist not of any one muscle, or set of muscles, but combine the wholesome activity of many.

In health these muscles are strong and active. Disease of the pelvic parts comes from their enfeebled condition or their habitual inaction.

The nutrition of muscles is stimulated by

action; they are made powerful by cautious and suitable exercise.

Timely repetitions of the process described, and others similar to it, would increase the nutrition and power of the muscles so engaged.

The action of *other* muscles might coöperate with them, and contribute to the same end. These, too, might be strengthened in a similar manner.

In this way, by calling into action and replenishing the power of the sustaining muscles, the whole convoluted digestive tube, including its inferior extremity, could be lifted up and maintained in the position which, through weakness of certain controlling elements, it had lost.

Cases of male adults, precisely similar to the one described, are not numerous.

But the female pelvis has certain *additional* contents, consisting of the generative intestine, the uterus and its appendages. These are perfectly analogous in location, and subject to the control of the same sustaining elements as those of the alimentary intestine.

The cases of affections of these organs in females are overwhelmingly numerous. Will these parts of the female obey the same restorative influences? To what extent does the cause of rectal prolapsus, now apparently demonstrated to consist of *unantagonized gravitation*, apply to a similar condition of the generative intestine? To determine the facts relating to this point seemed to be my prospective task.

The experiment above narrated, if experiment it may be called, plainly suggested a cause for female suffering additional to those commonly acknowledged; a cause very inadequately provided for—a cause to which those usually assigned are but *secondary*. Unantagonized, this cause is necessarily a preliminary to disease of the pelvic contents, not of any specified form, but of all forms which grow out of that constant element of disease—hyperæmia.

In the case described, the subsidence of the difficulty and the means which removed it were visible and unmistakable. The operation was simple, could be repeated an unlimited number of times, and would be available even in the most intractable case of the kind.

On the other hand, it is recorded experience that the usual remedial measures, however powerful, fall short of the purpose—are, in fact, palliative rather than curative, temporary rather than permanent.

The rationale of real cure of pelvic disorders was in this case apparent; the threshold had been approached; confirmation, derived from repeated practical success, was only wanting.

My patient received instructions for practicing several of the "movements" previously described, which were the suggestions of the moment. It was remarked and believed that the case was put in the patient's own hands. He practiced without help, following the examples I set him. He had no more difficulty. The rectum required no more to be replaced by digital manipulation, and in very short time required no attention.

The cure seemed too sudden to be real; he therefore, at my request, lingered a week or two for observation. No untoward symptoms supervening, he returned to his home *permanently*, as well as perfectly, restored from his prolonged and distressing complaint.

WEAK BOWELS OF CHILDREN.

Children of weakly and especially of strumous habits are more liable to the symptoms above described than men; and since the cure is very rapid, simple and complete, I will describe the process. Children do not object to any process that involves exercise applied to them, and they make excellent patients for this treatment.

To cause the prolapsed bowels of a child to recede to their place, the mother or nurse may lay it across her lap, face downward. Then she may separate her knees, so that the breast shall rest upon one knee, and the legs upon the other, in the meanwhile placing one hand upon the abdomen and the other upon the back of the child. Now press with both hands, but more with the *upper* hand, which will cause the body of the child to bend or become convex downward; next press more with the hand placed *under* the body, so as to cause the body to be in a line. At every alternate pressure of either hand the child is directed to straighten itself, with which action of the child the mother should so coöperate as to render it more complete and effective. This action may be repeated three or four times. The extruded bowel will return to its place as the direct result of the operation. To maintain and render permanent the advantage thus easily secured, it is necessary to repeat the movement two or three times daily. The abdomen should also receive a thorough kneading by the hand, while the child is lying either face or back downward.

These movements will be found not only to cure the existing condition, but to obviate any tendency of the bowel to pass down.

ELEVATION OF THE CONTENTS OF THE FEMALE PELVIS—GENERAL WEAKNESS AND PELVIC LAXITY—COMPLETE DISABILITY.

Having had repeated and incontestable demonstration that the digestive organs, including its lower extremity, are susceptible of being raised, and permanently retained in a more elevated position, and that the accomplishment of this constitutes a reliable cure in a distressing and intractable class of cases, I was anxious to carry forward the principles involved to a new and more extensive field.

The probabilities of achieving still wider and more important results were strengthened by such considerations as follow: The processes thus far employed required the action of but few of the sustaining muscles, and some of these but feebly. By having recourse to a variety of positions and processes, many other muscles might be put in action. All the muscles that could have anything to do directly or remotely with sustaining the abdomen, or communicating motion to it, could be successively set in vigorous action; and so the combined products of such action could be rendered available. The fundamental principle being established, could be carried out in part, or wholly, in a great variety of forms. The exigencies of different cases could be thus met. Other principles than that of sustentation, as, for instance, that of gravitation, could be made auxiliary to the same ends. Great delicacy and much tact could be employed in cases requiring these qualities. There was practically no limit to the power that was available, since it is self-regenerating. Ends are proportionate to means.

The feasibility of elevating and strengthening the contents of the pelvis had been fairly demonstrated. It now became a point of interest to determine the range of the applicability of this principle. Would it be available in cases of extreme weakness and helplessness? This inquiry was set at rest by the satisfactory issue of the following case:

A gentleman consulted me with reference to his wife's health, concerning which he gave this account: She had borne two children, and three years before had suffered a miscarriage. From the effects of this accident she had not recovered.

For the first two years she was able to stand and walk a few steps occasionally; but during the last year she had been confined to her bed. She had had the usual variety of advice in a city renowned for its physicians, but none of this afforded more than temporary alleviation. During the latter half of this period she wore a ring pessary. Her last physician caused her removal to the sea-shore, for the advantage of change of atmosphere. There she remained, as helpless, however, as before.

There appeared to be nothing mysterious about this case, except failure to recover. In what does the impediment to recovery essentially consist, is the problem to solve. She was young, without hereditary fault or constitutional tendency to disease. Evidently she ought not to remain ill; there is some reason not assigned in medical literature why such so remain. Medical practice displays no resources adequate to cope with the difficulties these cases present; it seems too poor to minister more than temporary relief, and it becomes apparently bewildered in the attempt to respond to the perpetual cry of symptoms. It is apt to forget that many of these are but finger boards, which, if we remove, we lose our way.

Thus it is, that in an endless variety and abundance of detail we often neglect the guidance of first principles.

The solution of the difficulty here presented appears to lie in this statement ;—the sustaining power is absent, and the necessary consequence, local hyperæmia, is present. The facts so patent ought to suggest this inquiry : Can muscles obtain increased power and renewed action while action, the first and most imperative need of the case, is practically denied? Give this action, however passively, and you contribute to this power. Not the mere chemical action of ordinary remedies, but absolute, dynamic force, the essential concomitant of all physiological activity. The thing needed is not the mere mechanical holding up of certain parts, even if it could be well done, for this would allow them to remain as hyperæmic and weak as before ; but active, variable, vital support.

It was feasible, in this instance, to give the husband such directions as would be likely to result in increasing the nutrition and power of certain muscles, and consequently help the parts in intimate relations therewith. In a month a good beginning had been made. The wife could now walk about her room several times a day, and was anxious to come under more specific treatment, better adapted to her special condition. For this, arrangements were accordingly made.

Having now personal supervision of the case, I removed the pessary, brought the sustaining muscles into action, and duly excited change of local capillary and interstitial fluids. This, it will be noticed, was previous to the attainment of that full and unequivocal certainty respecting these principles that is now possessed; and also before the invention of the facilities which have since been found so necessary to carry forward these principles to their greatest practical successes. With the simplest means, however, I had the gratification to see the patient improve with great rapidity. The uterus soon receded to its natural position; and the evidences of congestion at the same time disappeared. In two weeks she could walk, and even mount stairs with but little trouble, and with no unpleasant consequences. Her father, who kept close watch of her case and was abundantly solicitous of the result, had expressed his calculations that six months was a fair length of time in which to give what was then regarded a new remedy a proper trial. Feeling perfectly well, however, and further treatment relating to pelvic organs being regarded as superfluous, she returned home at the end of three weeks and engaged in the duties of her household. The restoration proved entirely permanent.

It is quite unfair to judge of the gravity of a disease by the facility with which it is restored. That would be begging the question. The probabilities are that this patient would have continued, like thousands of others, an invalid for an indefinite period, resisting the ordinary stereotyped resources. For, conceding all that is claimed for iron, quinine, strychnine and similar remedies, it is not claimed that the specially weak organs are strengthened by their use. It follows that the same inharmony in the distribution of nutrition prevails as before. The pelvic organs, both relatively and practically, are as weak as ever, and if any progress toward health be made, it is of a kind that does not satisfy the patient; she continues as hopeless and helpless as ever. Sooner or later, grave secondary pathological changes occur in the uterus and appendages, or in the spine, superinduced by continuous lying, or in the digestive organs, or in all these parts, which proportionally diminish the chances for a successful issue of the case.

Medical practice sometimes finds itself placed in this most singular predicament : It has abundant, excellent, inestimable remedies for all these *secondary* affections. To cure them would be easy, were it not for the *primary* one. It must be confessed that the value of such remedies is sadly compromised by the persistent obstinacy of this primary disease—the disease which causes the disease. The natural inference is, that the *cause* is still unaffected. The needs of the invalid—the indications of treatment for the primary disease—continue the same, and so long as ignored or neglected the invalid must remain an invalid.

XVI.

CHRONIC MENORRHAGIA.

THE result of treatment by strengthening processes proves that very diverse symptoms often depend on conditions very nearly alike. Great weakness and laxness of fibre with atony of the whole pelvic region will give rise to several other classes of symptoms, as well as those above described. One of them is hemorrhage. The actual difference between the condition of the uterus in the case last described and in a case of hemorrhage might be covered by the tip of the finger. Where hemorrhage is a symptom, the weakness or laxity allows exudation, or uncaps a vessel. The difference is hardly sufficient to justify the regarding of the latter as a distinct disease.

With these principles in view, the physician's therapeutic applications should not be so much controlled by what appears to be the leading symptom, as by the cause of its manifestation.

In chronic periodical hemorrhages this principle meets with apt illustration. The womb will not acquire contractile strength, while the general system remains lax. If there is too much flow *from* the womb, it is a pretty clear indication that there is too much flow *to* that organ. This flow to the womb will not be restrained by medical application; these can only affect the outflow. To check or restrain the outflow is not entirely relevant to the purpose. It disposes of a transient symptom, but has little to do with the condition on which that symptom depends. The treatment here discussed aims primarily to affect conditions. The symptom is sure to succumb with its cause. This treatment employs the blood to sustain the general powers of the body; which done, it cannot appear in injurious superabundance during the periodical discharge.

It is the practical trust in these principles which gives the opportunity for the demonstration of their correctness, and it is gratifying to present cases in which the evidences are indubitable. From many of this kind I will select the following:

A lady came under my care seven years after

the birth of her last child. For two years her monthly periods had extended through half, often more than half, the month, sometimes, indeed, allowing her no interval. The hemorrhage was usually alarming during the first few days, attended by fainting fits, and great physical and nervous prostration. During the intervals she was able to walk about the room, and sometimes to ride out, being always carried over the stairs. She was very pale; even her lips were always bloodless. She had received the usual course of topical and tonic treatment. This had probably ameliorated her condition, but withal she was gradually declining.

I adhered to my usual rule in this case, which is to make, at first, no topical applications, reserving these for a subsequent resource, if the need of such be demonstrated. In this case the result proved that there was no need of any local treatment whatever. There was considerable hemorrhage at the return of the first period, after she came under my charge, but its duration was shortened. For four months after this, during which she received treatment, the periods were perfectly natural and healthful, except one slight irregularity fully explained by emotional causes to which she was suddenly subjected.

It might be supposed by those who know nothing of the effects of the processes employed that they are forbidden in case of great prostration. This would be a mistake. These are the very cases where self-help is out of the question, for which the treatment is peculiarly applicable. It must be kept in mind that this treatment is subject to endless variations, and must always be adapted to the invalid's wants. When there is no power, none is required of the patient, and never is the strength unpleasantly tasked.

Within a year after the application of the treatment in the case above referred to, the patient was delivered of twins, without unusual hemorrhage, and made an easy and rapid recovery.

OBSTRUCTION OF THE CERVICAL CANAL FROM FLEXION.

The weakness of muscle, and the consequent deficient motion which is characteristic of all forms of pelvic affections, very easily gives origin to deformity. The unrestrained pressure of the overlying and the contiguous parts will cause the uterus to become bent by the position into which it is thus forced.

When the uterus deviates from its natural position, and its axis remains straight, it cannot justly be regarded as diseased. The affection belongs to those dominant parts which control its position. The location of the organ is subject to change, with the nature and degree of this control. It is hence this latter condition which demands rectification. The controlling muscles are the proper, and, in most cases, the only objects of treatment. Remedial applications to the womb in this case are not only unnecessary but prejudicial; their use betrays a lack of consideration of those interdependent relations which have been insisted on.

When, however, the womb becomes bent at the junction of its body with its neck, we have new symptoms depending on essentially the same causes. This condition of the womb requires more time and careful adjustment of means to effect restoration; still, the radical treatment is the successful one, and the ordinary remedial measures may, in general, be dispensed with. The new symptoms are those arising from obstructed menstrual flow. This sometimes occasions great pain; at other times it causes distention of the womb and of its vessels, and consequent hemorrhage, ordinarily very difficult to control.

Extreme pain at the monthly periods was the characteristic symptoms of a lady who had borne two children, the youngest of whom was seven years old. This symptom had increased for a number of years, until it was insupportable. She usually became unconscious at the commencement of the periods, and remained so for hours, sometimes for a day. For a year or two before I saw her the physician in charge had, in anticipation of the periods, habitually inserted a catheter through the cervical canal, extending it quite to the cavity of the womb. This precaution always proved effectual in preventing pain. The effect was obviously to straighten the canal and give egress to the secretion, preventing its accumulation and the consequent painful distention of the cavity of the womb, and thus quite obviating the cause of pain.

This lady presented a nervous, emaciated, worn appearance, and expressed herself as having a feeling of desperation. Pursuing the plan above indicated, I proceeded, *not* to turn or push up, or straighten, or make applications to the suffering organ, but to elevate the diaphragm and the whole mass of digestive organs, and to incite and extend downward the natural motions derived from respiration.

To accomplish these purposes I depended exclusively on the application of the processes already described. The methods usually employed were regarded as subsidiary at the best, and were reserved for the future, if needed. But they were never required. The processes for extending the motions of the diaphragm to the pelvis and for removing the superincumbent abdominal weight were extremely gratifying to her. She even introduced to her home some of the simplest mechanical conveniences in order to enjoy more fully their advantages.

Her monthly period recurred in three weeks after commencing the treatment, and *she experienced no pain whatever;* everything pertaining to the menstrual function was perfectly natural and easy.

This was the first time in many years that she had passed a menstrual period without severe pain, except when obviated by the catheter. Her general health, strength, appearance and spirits were all proportionally improved. At her next period, the catamenia were absent, and in due time a child was born to her. After her return to the menstrual state, she remained free from any menstrual difficulty.

In this case the relief from pain, and the severe nervous symptoms and reflex action which were its concomitants, was due to the changed position and shape of the womb. This latter effect was secured by removing its cause, which demonstrably was the interference and pressure of the superimposed digestive organs. This latter object it was impossible to accomplish by any treatment, from whatever source, applied to the uterus itself; that organ not being previously at fault, though suffering extremely, and causing suffering throughout the whole system.

HYPERTROPHY, GENERAL AND PARTIAL.

In most cases of chronic uterine affections there is an increase of substance and of weight either of some portion or the whole of the body, some portion or the whole of the neck, or the entire uterus. An examination of the affected part not only reveals the exact location and extent of change in the organs, but should also suggest to the reflective mind that this change is but the natural effect of prolonged hyperæmia. The swelling is due primarily to an accumulation of fluids in the affected part. These fluids distend the vessels and escape into the tissues surrounding them. This excess of nutrient material lodged in the part becomes, to some extent, organized, and incorporated with the normal tissues. Why one portion of the generative apparatus becomes the seat of disease rather than another, and why disease assumes the form of excessive discharges in one case and of retention with swelling in another, is beyond the present knowledge of medical science, and we must be content with the plain facts as they present themselves to our observation and experience.

But nothing is more reasonable than to presume that the main and efficient cause is the same in either case, and that the particular form of the effect may be determined by some intermediate though unrecognized circumstance. The difference in the two cases would appear to be, that in the one, material is injuriously discharged, and in the other, it is injuriously retained, the essential fact being excess of material—hyperæmia in the pelvis. The cause of the hyperæmic condition has been sufficiently considered in previous chapters. The remedial endeavor is to dispose of the superfluous material, which is at once the evidence and the effect of disease.

But just as truly as in malposition from superincumbent weight, as in menorrhagia, as in ulceration and leucorrhœa, as in dysmenorrhœa from congestion or occlusion, hypertrophy, the product of the hyperæmic condition, is not self-sustaining, but will certainly disappear with its cause. Correct practice, it seems to me, should make its first attack on this cause, whether the mere effect be treated or not. There will be plenty of time to remedy the effect, but no time should be lost in remedying the cause.

It is for this condition that local remedial applications are in favor with many physicians. If judiciously managed, such applications may diminish surplus local fluids, and even solids. These objects are gained by the power of such remedies to increase local absorption or by a temporary increase of discharges through the vaginal outlet. The physician avows his theory of the process of cure by his selection of remedies.

As in the cases already cited, the use of such remedies may be proper as palliatives, but they are incompetent to fulfil the radical indications. Abundant cures are reported, and doubtless occur, even under the exclusive use of local treatment; but it is not quite fair, therefore, to bestow on it all the credit of restoration. Nature, unaided, is always working for this end. Improved hygiene, secured either by accident or design, should have its share of credit. Let local applications have their proper place as temporary expedients whose best results must inevitably and necessarily fall short of the requirements of these cases. The need obviously is, not merely to overcome the morbid local conditions, but to obviate the tendency to such conditions—the accumulation of superfluous material affording a nidus for morbid change.

It cannot be too strenuously insisted on by the physician, or too deeply impressed on the mind of the patient, that there are two factors to be considered in every case of pelvic disease, and that only one of these factors is pelvic. The other is equally indispensable to the existence of such disease. It consists in the support afforded to the disease by the system. But for this factor, which is usually overlooked by all parties, there could be no local disease to medicate. To withhold the support of disease is to secure health, as withholding fuel is to extinguish fire. This is a therapeutic consideration of first importance.

The reason why frequent repetitions of local applications are necessary is now apparent. The causative process is constant, and is not abated by such treatment; the restorative process must be equally constant, or no permanent ground is gained. Two distinct aims of treatment are recognized; one is that of removing the cause of disease, which can almost always be done, and when thoroughly effected there will be no recurrence of the malady; and the other aim is chiefly palliative, and is confined for the most part to the consequences of disease,—its local manifestation.

We can now assign to the local and the radical treatment their relative values, and will be able to judge which is the principal and which the auxiliary treatment, when both are at the same time employed.

It is an incorrect supposition that local medical applications for hypertrophy are the only curative recourse. They are neither the surest nor most rapid processes for removing enlargements. Many physicians reject such remedies, preferring to rely on constitutional and specific remedies. The action of rapid vibratory motion,* applied to the affected part and to the surrounding region, produces absorption and the reduction of enlargement in a remarkable and far more satisfactory degree. Scrutiny of the methods and effects of this process will be found highly instructive to all interested in therapeutic inquiries.

If topical applications are to be made, I decidedly prefer, as before stated, the milder rather than the more chemically potent remedies.

Remedies selected from the former class are capable of influencing vital processes to a far

* The reader is referred to a communication in the Medical Record for Nov. 15, 1870, "On Vibration as a Mechanical Influence in Promoting Capillary Circulation," by A. F. A. King, M. D.; also to articles by the author in the New York Medical Journal for November, 1869, and April, 1870.

greater extent than the latter, and therefore make a more profound curative impression. Every physician of experience has his favorite remedies and methods. For such applications I have found glycerine to be a convenient and excellent vehicle for conveying the medicament to the seat of the affection. With a proper syringe and the requisite dexterity, from one-fourth to one-half a drachm of the solution may be applied to the lining of the cervical canal, or even the metrial cavity, if desirable. Glycerine spreads itself well over the membrane, and detaches any tenacious adherent secretion, and its osmotic qualities insure the absorption of the medicament in sufficient amount to impress and guide the vital action of the part. This impression extends to the subjacent tissues as well as to the lining of the cavities. It is important that the piston-rod of the syringe be accurately marked, so that the physician shall know the precise amount of the fluids used; the pipe should also be similarly marked in half-inches so as to be determined by the touch, in order to know precisely to what point the medicament is applied. It is better if the orifice at the end of the pipe be stopped and others made at its sides near the end, the better to distribute the application.

I cannot presume to dictate to others what drugs should be employed in this manner to meet different emergencies. The selection of remedies must be governed not only by the physician's ideas of the local affection he has to deal with, the temperament and idiosyncrasies of his patient, but also by his breadth of acquaintance and familiarity with the materia medica, which undergoes constant expansion.

XVII.

HYPERTROPHY AND RETROFLEXION.

There are causes acting outside of and upon the uterus which coöperate to bend its upper portion over and backward, thus producing incurvation. Among these may be numbered the following:

The pessary supplies an upward resistance, antagonizing the weight of the superior organs. The uterus is thus compressed between two opposing forces, and must therefore become bent in some direction, usually backward.

Exterior supporters press strongly upon the lower portion of the abdomen, and bend the uterus backward.

Closely fitting garments press the abdominal contents dōwn and upon the uterus, bending it backward.

The effect of all compression upon the abdomen is to give a backward direction to the line of all motion affecting the viscera. Instead of such motion being parallel with the spine, and hence directed to the front of the pelvis, it corresponds more nearly with the curve of the sacrum, and pushes the uterus down under its promontory. The condition of the uterus after confinement or miscarriage is particularly favorable for the above-named causes to become operative. The weight of its upper portion aids the causes named.

The chief cause, it will be seen, is identical with that which has been presented as the cause of the other forms of affection of the pelvic contents—the lack of restraining power over the visceral weight. In the present case the cause affects the uterine mass; in those previously referred to it affected the uterine circulation, nutrition and nerves.

The first impression regarding cases of this kind is that mechanical assistance is demanded; that by means of the curved sound the womb should be raised to its proper place and straightened. But the result of experience with this procedure is far from satisfactory. The organ will neither be persuaded nor compelled by this operation to remain in the place thus assigned it. And why should it, against the pressure of the visceral mass, which has not in the least been changed?

Disease of the rectum, as well as constipation, is a frequent concomitant of retroversion. This is an almost necessary consequence of the close proximity into which the parts are brought, and from the fact that both organs are affected by a common cause. The necessary straining at stool, the inevitable use of aperient medicines and injections, and the direct pressure caused by the womb upon the tissues of the rectum, conspire to produce rectal disease.

Retroversion, with its effects both upon the uterus and rectum, is, however, quite removable on the principles herein inculcated. The first impression produced by the elevating movements may appear inconsiderable; but the effects gather strength by repetition, and the desired end is in due time secured.

Very debilitated cases must first be treated with reference to the development of the supporting muscles, and the other conditions that have been specified as required for uterine support and health; for all endeavors to secure sustentation, in the absence of these, are fruitless and discouraging. These muscles, even in the weakest, may be thus fructified by well-directed manipulations, stretchings, rubbings, with moderate and well-timed demands on the voluntary powers.

After the strength, and therefore the sustaining power, has thus been acquired, it is not a difficult matter to apply it to the desired use; and such movements may now be easily employed as will progressively, and with great certainty, restore the uterus to its proper position, where it will be permanently sustained.

In cases where treatment has from some cause been suspended before restoration was complete, it has been observed to go on spontaneously to perfection, thus demonstrating the power as well as relevancy of the means employed. A good illustration of these principles will be found in the following instance: A lady was placed under my care by the physician who had attended her with unsatisfactory results for several years. She had been reared with the utmost tenderness, every want having been anticipated by wealthy and indulgent parents. This, it must be conceded, is not the way to develop a sound and robust constitution. After marriage she bore four children in rapid succession. Her physical powers broke down under responsibilities to which she was inadequate. She became pale, thin, weak and nervous to the last degree. She had been in this state for the last two years. She was unable to leave her room without assistance, and made the journey to me under the influence of strong stimulants. An examination revealed a greatly enlarged and retroverted womb, the neck thickened and os eroded, and affording a profuse leucorrhœa. Evacuations of the bowels, whether obtained by the aid of aperients or enemas, were performed with the greatest difficulty, and followed by prolonged prostration. Great tenderness of the coccyx compelled her, when sitting, always to use an air cushion. Added to these symptoms was extreme depression of spirits, which, unfortunately, were seriously aggravated by domestic causes.

Having but little muscular fibre, or indeed other fleshy covering for her frame, the treatment could only be administered, at first, in a very delicate manner. Increase of muscular nutrition, and the consequent diminishing of nervous activity and suffering, were the great points to be secured. A resisting quality—hardness of fibre—was also to be developed in every part of the body. A winter's treatment was so far effective as to restore quiet and comfort; to enable her to walk about, even in the street, without difficulty; to mitigate the rectal obstruction so far as to allow spontaneous evacuations of the bowels; to reduce considerably the size of the womb, and enable her to sit in the ordinary way without discomfort. The retroversion was much improved, but not entirely corrected.

After her return to her home in another city I continued to hear of her improving health. I saw her three or four years later, and found the retroversion entirely overcome. She was enjoying very comfortable health. She had received no other remedial treatment in the meantime, but had strictly followed the instructions I had given her. It is evident that the change of position had been wrought by rendering effective the dominant physiological elements. They had continued to acquire strength until muscular preponderance was attained. This effect tended to increase, because the nutritive activities of these supporting muscles had been specially strengthened.

In the above case, the extreme anæmic condition was a serious obstacle to recovery. The following, its opposite, verging upon plethora, afforded equal disadvantages to be overcome by the treatment. This lady had been married eight years, without children. Her illness commenced with a severe, acute disease, terminating in metritis, which was continued in a chronic form. After lingering in a nearly helpless condition for several months, she was brought to me for treatment. There was great hypertrophy of the uterus, and its fundus pressed strongly against the rectum, passages from the bowels being obtained with the greatest difficulty. There was much chronic cellulitis also present. She was very fleshy, the organs were closely compacted, and I found it impossible to change the position of the uterus in the least by manipulation. The difficulties in the way of restoring the uterus to its natural position were in this case extreme, and it was only by waiting the effects of appropriate movements that it could be hoped for. Improvement, however, went perceptibly on; local sensitiveness passed away, the uterus diminished in size, and again became mobile, and the general health and strength gradually returned. After three months she had so far recovered as to return to her home and her usual household duties. A year and a half afterwards she gave birth to her first child.

Following is an account of a severe case of retroversion, much complicated by the effects of topical treatment. This lady had borne several children, and had enjoyed uninterrupted health previous to the present affection. For four or five years increasing symptoms of retroversion had been manifested, such as obstinate constipation, difficulty in relieving the bowels, followed by great nervous prostration, etc. The latter portion of this time constipation had been absolute, relieved only by aperients and injections with much effort. Her family physician failing to remove the difficulty, she came to New York for advice, and placed herself under the care of one of our ablest and most renowned uterine specialists. She had several terms of receiving treatment, the last of which continued seven months. The treatment fully represented the resources at the command of those who give exclusive attention to this branch of medical practice, and are its acknowledged exponents. A portion of the treatment consisted in the injection into the uterine cavity of various medicaments, among which chromic acid was several times applied. These applications required confinement to the bed for ten or twelve days, to await the subsidence of the inflammation, and the passing away of the slough produced by the destructive effect of the caustic.

In the present instance, however, there was, following these applications, no such increase of discharges as would indicate the passing away of the parts destroyed by the applications. Other symptoms, located in the rectum, now revealed themselves. A yellowish white, thick, tenacious discharge from the bowels appeared daily or oftener. This discharge was often bloody, resembling dysenteric discharges, and was seldom mixed with the alvine evacuations; the amount varied from a drachm to an ounce. Examinations and consultations were had with reference to this discharge, but no relief, much less cure, was obtained. She returned to her home not in the least improved, but with the addition of the rectal disease. A few weeks subsequently she placed herself under my care.

The first thing to be done was to remove a very large metallic pessary, the third that had been inserted, of increasing sizes. The os uteri was so high in front as scarcely to be reached; the fundus was much enlarged, and pressed firmly against the rectum and sacrum. By the aid even of combined rectal and vaginal touch, and the advantage of the semi-prone position, but slight change in the position of the uterus could be effected.

To carry upward and forward the fundus of the womb, and to keep it in this new position, reliance was placed solely on the operations described in the foregoing pages. Once only was the sound employed to turn forward the fundus of the womb, and this not till it had become evident that the condition of the abdominal and chest muscles had undergone such radical change that the cause, so far as it consisted in unantagonized gravitation, had been removed. The morbid discharges from the rectum gradually diminished from the first—not, however, without their having one or two periods of aggravation by causes that were readily accounted for in temporary disturbances of health. At the end of two months these discharges had wholly ceased; the action of the bowels, in the meantime, having become perfectly regular and natural. The mouth of the womb had returned to its natural position, and the fundus was no longer found pressing against the rectum. Several months after discontinuing the treatment there had been no return of previous symptoms. During the term of treatment she was permitted to ascend and descend stairs, and since then she has exerted herself without restraint and without the least detriment.

The rectal affection followed so directly and closely upon the intra-uterine medication as to leave no reasonable doubt that it resulted from this treatment. Once established, it proved incurable till its secondary causes—namely, the intrusion of the uterus, and the irritation of frequent ineffectual strainings in defecation, conjoined with pelvic hyperæmia, which always exists in such cases—were removed.

In the case above cited, two distinct therapeutic principles were brought to a direct practical test. The one restricts itself to what efficacy may be derived from local treatment; for though general tonics and alteratives may be employed, no practical advantage is gained by their prolonged administration. The other considers the pelvic affection, however complicated and severe, to be referable to certain specific and easily understood deficiencies, quite removed from the pelvis.

The one is content with therapeutic measures which have their beneficial uses; but a preposterous degree of importance is attached to those measures which, after prolonged experience, have proved inadequate to produce radically curative effects. The other, conceding the utility of those measures so far as their province extends, not only demonstrates their insufficiency, but supplies direct and unequivocally curative means.

Common sense inquires:

Are the natural supports of the uterus strengthened by artificial sustentation of that organ?

Does muscular power increase by repression or by use?

Is local congestion removed by attracting the bodily fluids to the congested region?

Are the products of local congestion and inflammation most readily removed while the cause of local obstruction remains?

What becomes of the soluble products of potent chemicals with organic matter when confined in contact with mucous membrane?

Metallic salts being thus introduced into the

system, what are the evidences of their cumulative effects?

Can the circulation and nutrition of a helpless invalid be best promoted while she is deprived of the most common and simple conditions of health?

If the uterus is in health sufficiently provided with supports, why not allow the same for invalids?

If the uterus becomes hypertrophied, why not divert the circulation from it?

Why not continue to the weak organs the same vivifying agencies that exist in health?

If the pelvic and vaginal tissues are lax and feeble, why stretch them inordinately by instruments?

If the uterus becomes bent from the overlying pressure, why supply an upward counterpressure? Why not remove the superincumbent weight, and allow the suffering organ to recede to its place?

Why is *common sense* out of place in matters pertaining to health more than in other matters? Should a recognition of a few of the facts of pathology be entitled to equal regard with the recognition of many?

XVIII.

SECONDARY EFFECTS OF MEDICAL APPLICATIONS TO THE UTERUS.

Medical literature abounds in discussions upon the subject of the successive stages of disease, the sequelæ of disease, the secondary specific diseases, etc. It would be well if the indirect and remote effects of remedies were also made the subject of special investigation; for there is good reason to believe that the direct and immediate effects are but a portion, in some cases but a small portion, of these consequences, and were all the facts elicited, they would, in many cases, greatly modify our therapeutics.

It scarcely admits of dispute that the remedial effects of drugs are intimately connected with their capacity to produce abnormal effects if used in larger quantity. These are immediate effects, and are generally admitted to pass rapidly away with the producing cause, through the channels by which matters are discharged from the system. But these are not the effects to which I refer.

It is the consequences of continued and prolonged use of remedies to which I desire to call attention. Even the most volatile, as alcohol, it is well known, makes a permanent and often ineradicable impression on the nervous system. Many other things in common use, possessing drug and semi-drug characteristics, produce such effects on the nerves as to demand their constant repetition—not, however, because of any nutritive quality they yield. The principle involved is explained on the supposition of the existence of a more or less permanent affinity in the material thus used for some element of nerve-substance.

When drugs consist of substances which have a decided and demonstrable affinity for some tissue, the probability of cumulative and permanent results from their use is much increased. Metallic compounds, as oxides, chlorides, etc., belong to this class. These substances enter into chemical union with the connective and perhaps other tissues possessing low vitality. The well-known effects of the compounds of lead, whether introduced into the system by accident, as in the use of water from lead pipes or in the case of painters, or by design, as in its use for face and head washes, affords testimony on this point. The salts of zinc, arsenic, silver, and many others having metallic basis, have been proved to possess analogous affinities. We have seen the peculiar specific effects of chromic acid in the case last related. The history of the case supports the view that the neutralized compound of the acid with organic substance was absorbed, to be physiologically eliminated. The excess of eliminatory material, however, converted the physiological into a pathological process, which withstood ordinary remedies.

That the silver salts have an affinity for some constituent of nerve-substance is supported by the fact that they have acquired a reputation as remedial in some forms of nerve disease; but the probability of pathological effects arising from frequent applications of nitrate of silver has scarcely been entertained. It has been asserted that the compound of this salt with organic substances is insoluble, and therefore harmless. This insolubility has been assumed without sufficient warrant. The fluids of the body are pervaded by chloride of sodium, which is quite capable of decomposing and effecting the solution of silver compounds, thus rendering them capable of exerting their specific influence.

The fact which has been stated, that prolonged treatment of women by local applications renders them liable to recurring attacks of pelvic neuralgia, is also in point. The frequent absorption of small quantities of medicaments would be quite likely to render the nerves sensitive, as the first pathological effect. But pelvic neuralgia may be referred to other causes, and the one above assigned be regarded as insufficient. Yet stronger evidence of this effect is not wanting. In three instances lately under my care, where these remedies had been freely employed, the prolonged local treatment was followed by great neuralgia of the extremities, terminating in partial paralysis. This result accords with the known effect of the drugs. It also leads to the surmise that if such cases as sciatica, paralysis, and other nervous disorders, were investigated with reference to the kind and amount of medicines employed, much interesting and instructive truth would be elicited.

UTERINE COMPLICATED WITH SPINAL AFFECTIONS.

A characteristic evidence of uterine affections is pain in the back—sometimes in the lumbar region, sometimes in the sacral, generally in the cervical. The upright position, whether walking or standing, gives rise to this pain. There is hence a great disinclination to this position; it is assumed only when necessity compels. The ability to take this position gradually diminishes, since unused muscles are poorly nourished. To the existence of pain is soon and certainly added the lack of power. This stage of the disease having arrived, the patient habitually assumes the recumbent position, from which it is with the utmost difficulty she is reclaimed, if, indeed, she be reclaimed at all.

A cursory glance at anatomy and physiology will show the connection between the back and the pelvis, and explain why pelvic affections are indicated by symptoms referable to the back.

When the uterus and appendages suffer disease, in almost any of the forms to which they are liable, they often become abnormally sensitive, resembling in this particular other parts of the body. Sensation is painfully awakened by locomotion, since the actions of lifting, twisting, and the like, of the lower limbs are well calculated to disturb the contents of the pelvis. The causes of such disturbance are hence instinctively avoided, and walking, etc., suspended.

But the spine itself often becomes seriously affected. This is owing to several causes. One is, the capacity for sensation which resides in the spinal cord is abnormally and continuously excited. Pelvic disorders afford a constant supply of sensorial impressions. This tends to increase the nutrition and power of the cord, as all powers are strengthened by exercise, whether normal or abnormal. Hyperæmia of the cord is the ultimate result of the constant operation of this cause.

Another cause of spinal complication with pelvic disease is the mesenteric connection in the vicinity of the lumbar region—a connection which supplies sensory nerves to the abdominal contents. In the lax condition of the abdominal walls that co-exist with pelvic affections this connection is tasked with aiding the support of the pendant mass. This fact may explain a portion of the lumbar pain and weariness almost invariably experienced by invalids of this kind.

Still another cause of the spinal complication is the effect of the habitual lying position that these invalids are compelled to assume. In proportion to the weakness is the laxity of the capillary spinal vessels. Much lying on the back, in connection with the heat thus confined in that portion of the body, favors this laxity and distension of the calibre of the vessels. This position also favors the gravitation of the circulating fluids toward the back, since, when lying, the back is the lowest part of the body, and in the absence of vigor of circulation the fluids yield to the law of gravitation. This still further distends the vessels of the spine and increases the congestion. The effect of much lying is even exhibited in the substance of the bones. They become soft and spongy, as has been proved by comparison of those from persons who have not, with those who have, subjected them to much use.

In health, the most powerful as well as the most reliable of all the aids to the circulation of the blood consists in ordinary exercise. When this is omitted or materially diminished, as it is in pelvic affections, the circulatory vessels are also badly nourished and become non-contractile—a state which highly favors congestion of any part which is inclined thereto from other causes.

The upright position demands the active use of all the muscles of the back to sustain the position. This secures their nutrition. They otherwise become shrunken, weak and powerless. The muscles of the back have an indispensable use besides that of maintaining their own power. *The action of these muscles serves as a necessary counterpoise to the action of the spinal cord.* While acting they receive blood, and in some degree withdraw it from the cord. It is in many cases possible to engage these muscles in action, with the effect of relieving the pain in the back and permanently removing its hyperæsthesia. This, however, is to be attempted only with the full understanding of the proper methods of procedure, and a due estimate of the invalid's condition. The ordinary action of spinal muscles in health prevents spinal congestion; their prescribed and cultivated action cures spinal congestion.

That exercise is the most powerful as well as reliable aid to the circulation is as true in disease as in health. But exercise does not necessarily imply exertion. It is here again that the principle of gravitation, which has been studied in another connection, becomes beneficent. If the body but change its position, the vessels upon which the hydrostatic pressure of the blood is exercised are also changed. Thus the vessels of every part of the body of a helpless invalid may be in succession exercised. The circulation may receive incalculable aid simply by frequent changes of position. Hence the lying position is not in the least a bar to the hopeful aid of exercise.

From these statements it is apparent that, on theoretic grounds, the tendency to spinal congestion should not only be obviated but even removed by suitable exercises. The difficulty consists in their adaptation and practical application. Ordinary exercises have already been proved not merely harmful but impossible. This fact is usually the first evidence of the existence of the affection.

The remedial advantages that may be derived from suitable exercises not having been properly investigated, there is, consequently, an absence of principle, rule or tact in the prescribing of these means. The objection that in unregulated quantities and kinds they become harmful lies equally against other remedies, and would exclude them all. This matter of adaptation and regulation, so as to adjust means to ends, forms the basis of success with this as with every other curative agent.

A good exemplification of the working of the principles above advanced was in the case of a recent patient. This lady's ill health began soon after the birth of a child, now eight years old. For the greater part of the intervening period she had maintained the recumbent position. She had received almost constant treatment for uterine disease.

She wore both a pessary and external supporter, and felt unable to do without either. She could walk a little on level ground, but could not ascend even a single step. She had a constant backache, increased by every effort with the legs. This precluded nearly all exertion.

The pessary was removed at the first, but it required persuasion, not much short of coercion, to induce her to lay aside the outside supporter. This, however, was soon accomplished.

There was an abundant and fetid leucorrhœal discharge, which required vaginal injections of chlorate of potash, with a little carbolic acid. Her treatment consisted in the application of the principles elucidated in this work.

Though very depressed in spirits, and hopeless of recovery—a natural consequence of her continually disappointed efforts—yet she made good progress, with no untoward symptoms supervening. In this case I made particular observation of the ascent of the womb in the pelvic cavity. It reached a position at least one and a half inches higher in the pelvis than that at which it was maintained by the pessary.

As is usual in these cases, the pelvic symptoms yielded to the treatment much more readily than those referable to the back. In five or six weeks she was able to mount two or three flights of stairs. In about three months she returned to her home, relieved of all her suffering, and able to engage in the active duties of life.

This case exhibits in a decided and just light the folly of attempting uterine sustentation by means of mechanical supporters. Even if these instruments really serve the purpose expected of them, no substantial good is effected; they have not supplied what was lacking; the same weakness of fibre, laxity of tissue and vessel, and sensitiveness of nerve prevails as before. On the contrary, much harm has frequently been wrought by their use. The blood has been attracted to rather than from the pelvic region, and it has been made the centre of nerve irritation and the focus of thought and feeling; and more than all —because the cause of all—the action of the sustaining muscular elements has been effectually repressed. Whatever improvement may occur during the use of these appliances is generally in spite of rather than in consequence of their use.

Such results of the applications of these principles as are detailed in this work ensue only from their judicious and careful employment. The heterogeneous and indiscriminate use of even these processes will not only fail of good results, but will work mischief. There must be clear and definite aims on the part of both physician and patient, or the means will be likely to be incongruous, and therefore fall short of the desired end.

XIX.

CONNECTION OF NERVOUS WITH PELVIC DISEASE.

It is popularly as well as professionally understood that what are called diseases of women are not confined to the organs within the pelvis, and that the effects of such diseases permeate throughout the body, exhibiting special and often disastrous consequences in the nervous system. This complication of nervous with pelvic disorder demands our attentive consideration, from the fact that it is often regarded as affording a key to the therapeutics of the nervous symptoms. While these symptoms are supposed to have their origin in the pelvis, they will naturally be medicated through the pelvis.

This, in my opinion, does not embrace a full understanding of the relations of these two classes of affections. Their co-existence is insufficient evidence of their co-relation. Their inter-dependence often extends no farther than community of origin; and they do not always sustain the relation of cause and effect which is wont to be attributed to them. This being the case, the treatment which is administered on the theory of such relationship falls far short of its purpose.

There is, indeed, a significant uniformity in the results of ordinary treatment of the two classes of affections. They exhibit the same intractability, and are confessedly equally difficult of removal, and they are apt to be treated with less regard to removal of causes than of symptoms. Radical causes being neglected in either case, the two forms of disease are treated with equal irrelevancy. When nervous maladies are connected with their true causes, more rational, and therefore radical, treatment will be available, and these affections will lose their hopelessness.

The ultimate cause of these nervous complications with pelvic affections is demonstrably identical with that of the pelvic affection. This cause may be stated as consisting of the *prolonged unequal distribution of functional activities.* Disuse and weakness of muscle are followed by other and not less serious consequences than disease of the pelvic contents. Restraint of muscular nutrition causes excess of that of nerve centres. This allows the nerve centres, which preside over sensation, emotion, and even the intellect, to monopolize the greater proportion of nutritive action, and therefore to engage in disproportionate and unrestrained activity. This unbalanced action in the various departments of the nervous system is the essential disease to which reference is now made.

These facts afford a distinct view of the nature and the relations of these two forms of diseased manifestation. Pelvic disease occurs because of insufficient muscular action, and power to maintain the organs in place and to properly circulate the blood. Local disease is the ultimate product of these failures. Nervous disease occurs as another effect of the same cause. The energies to which the system gives rise not being expended in their legitimate channels, through the muscles, must therefore seek the only remaining channels of expenditure, the nerves, and these, consequently, become morbidly active.

It is important to keep in view a leading principle of physiology, heretofore referred to. This is, that *all* force of which the bodily organs are the medium is the product of nutritive change in the organ, or at least the physiological department to which the force is referred. The quality of the power exhibited depends *directly* on the quality of the nutritive change whereby it is evolved. But it also depends *indirectly* upon the relation sustained by any form or mode of expression to other modes.

It follows that *pain, uncontrolled emotion,* and *mental introversion* are as truly methods of expression of the forces evolved by the system as are *agreeable sensations, recreation, exercise,* etc.

But the amount of force generated by the system is *limited.* It cannot produce more than a certain amount in health, while in disease the amount is always much restricted. It necessarily follows that excess of its expression through any one channel—that is, through the activity of any function—involves its diminution through other channels, or even, in some cases, its entire suspension.

This is equivalent to saying that one form of force may displace, partly or wholly, other forms. Consequently, the excessive action of any function is antagonistic to the welfare of other departments of the body.

This want of harmony, or coördination in the expression of force by the system, is functional disease. The other phenomena and phases of disease on the planes of chemistry, physiology, pathological anatomy, &c., may, for the present, be neglected. The evidences of the displacement of one form of bodily power by another, and of its healthful by its diseased expression, are found in such facts as these :

A neuralgic limb or muscle withers as inevitably as a paralyzed one. This indicates that the nutritive supply previously used in replenishing muscle is now employed to support the activity of those spinal centres which afford the morbid forces.

A person suffering pain is indisposed to action —has little power to employ in action. Her total power may remain the same, but it is otherwise directed. While so much activity is transpiring in spinal centres which is cognizable as pain, but little force remains subservient to the will to stimulate the muscles and to oppose external obstacles.

The strong exercise of the emotions, especially that morbid form known as hysteria, is followed by fatigue and evidences of exhaustion of power as certainly and quickly as violent muscular exercise.

The products of waste flowing from the body in these pathological states afford evidence of increased change of matter—retrograde metamorphosis—as indubitable as any physiological action.

The invalid who fixes and continues her attention upon an internal part, reverses its natural direction. The result proves that she inevitably becomes weaker, falls into a state of helplessness, and thus continues till circumstances restore the natural direction of nervous energy. In this case also, force is diverted from its normal channels, and is consequently misemployed.

The principle here stated has always been largely adopted in therapeutics. The employment of counter-irritation and revulsion, of which the internal as well as the external use of remedies furnish numerous illustrations, corroborate this statement. But the most complete and satisfactory evidence of all is the direct and practical test: *If muscles and connective tissue be rendered mechanically active, the pain previously suffered in the region ceases.* The new excitement in the muscles suppresses the morbid excitement of the nerve. This fact, which may be easily tested by corroborative experiment, affords evidence that the morbid and redundant forces evolved by the nerve centres has assumed another form. It becomes in the muscle dynamic power. This change is coincidental with the transfer of blood from one order of tissue to the other; and also with the repression and reduplication of cell life in the respective tissues from which the two forms of force emanate.

In discussing the diseases of the pelvic organs, it was shown that the cause was easily and directly traceable to imperfect muscular power and action. It now appears that the repression of muscular power and action is a necessary concomitant of excited and morbid nervous power. The conclusion is plain and direct, that a common cause is equally competent to produce both effects.

The forms which morbid innervation assumes correspond with the functions of the several portions of the nervous system. For convenience, they may be classified under the heads of *morbid sensation,* including both *hyperæsthesia* and *anæsthesia; morbid emotion,* including the various forms of *hysteria;* and *morbid intellection,* or unbalanced mental activity.

MORBID SENSATION.

The more common instances of the connection of pelvic with nervous disease are those cases which suffer much neuralgic pain, generally with the accompaniment of acute sensibility. This pain in different women assumes diverse forms, and may affect any portion of the body. But it has its favorite seats, the most prominent and characteristic of which is in the region of the pelvis. The next locality in importance is the back and loins. One side generally suffers much more than the other, especially in front of one hip. This frequently gives rise to the suggestion of ovarian disease, which suggestion is often rendered the more probable by fullness in the iliac region; but the result proves, in most cases, that these latter symptoms are due to other causes than these here mentioned. The neuralgic pain extends up the spine and down the legs, and the head generally suffers much.

When this neuralgic condition has been severe and prolonged, it is not uncommon for the muscles of the painful parts to show indications of retraction. One leg sometimes becomes permanently bent at the knee or hip, or both.

There is usually disorder of the digestive system, shown most frequently in capricious appetite and sluggishness of the bowels; the discharges are followed by nervous depression, continuing for several hours.

The uterine symptoms in these cases are usually confined to the more common evidences of metrial congestion, such as uterine and vaginal catarrh, and more or less marked anteversion. There may also be irregularities of the menstrual function, but no one type is more probable than another.

The condition of the muscular system furnishes a symptom no less conspicuous than the pain, and in entire consonance with preceding statements. The muscles of the whole body are feeble, lax, soft, and inactive. The patient is usually pale and thin. This is not, however, invariable; but plumpness is not a criterion of muscle. There are instances in which a good amount of fat covers a frame strung with small, feeble and inactive muscles. Of two cases now under my care, and nearly alike as regards the leading symptoms, one is extremely pale and bloodless, with thin weak muscles, while the other is florid and fleshy, but with flesh composed of only a small amount of muscle. This is apparent to the touch of one accustomed to examine invalids, as well as from the patient's inability to perform muscular tasks. The muscular deficiency is quite concealed by the adipose covering. These cases sometimes suffer injustice from uncharitable friends, who judge from apparent rather than actual conditions of health.

Accepting the principle that a relative increase of muscular action and nutrition tends to diminish that of the nerves, by withdrawing their nutrition, it is found to be a most difficult one to put in practice. It is, in fact, impracticable, without professional aid.

Muscular action (of the ordinary kind) begins with *effort*, which is action of the instruments of the will. This is confessedly *nervous* action, necessarily involving nerve centres, and requiring nutritive supply. The effect of this is, manifestly, to aggravate the previously existing diseased condition. But this effect it is the duty of the physician to prevent. Experience has taught him that exertion in any form may be and is likely to be prejudicial. Hence, not only is the invalid allowed to obey the instincts inseparable from inactive muscle—which is to avoid action—but she is constantly cautioned against putting forth efforts of any kind. Indeed, invalids date their ill health from over-doing, a thing most easily done when muscles are defective in power. Over-doing simply means *over-effort*—excessive nerve rather than muscular action. It is measured by changes wrought and suffered within the system, rather than what is accomplished exterior to it. These inconsequent efforts are followed by an aggravation of all the unpleasant symptoms, prolonged prostration, and great discouragement.

Ordinary exercise is prejudicial in these cases because it falls short of its purpose. It begins in nerve centres, and as the impulse or stimulus thus generated is not received by muscles, it must end in the same centres. The force is not diffused through the system and extended to objects beyond it, but is reflected back and precipitated upon parts unable to bear it.

The principle here unfolded receives daily practical illustrations. The following case shows the adverse effect of ill-advised efforts to carry the principle of exercise into practice for curative purposes. A young lady, of slight appearance and nervous temperament from childhood, had enjoyed good health until she broke down under the severe mental discipline of a boarding school which had made no provision for physical exercise. She returned from school weak, nervous, and dispirited. The common interests of life proved a burden to her; great fatigue followed every exertion. Her appetite was extremely poor and sleep very uncertain. Menstruation became irregular, scanty and painful; pain and tenderness appeared in the right side in front of the hip. Her disease was diagnosed uterine, and she was medicated accordingly for a year. She became more sensitive, the whole side becoming affected, and was confined to her room most of the time, when she came under my care. The improvement immediately following the application of the principles I have stated was rapid. In one month her pains had nearly vanished, and she could walk and ride with advantage. She was now prevailed upon to receive what purported to be the same treatment at home, with the addition of a little medication. Under this arrangement her pain returned and rapidly increased, the right side became intensely sensitive, and she was prostrated in bed, where she remained several months, her life being considered in danger during the latter part of this period. In this condition she was returned to me. There was excessive hyperæsthesia, and the right leg was spasmodically retracted at both the knee and hip joints. In this state the selection of successful methods of applying treatment (which was confined to manipulation, in accordance with the before-mentioned principles) was exceedingly difficult. So great was the prostration and the preponderance of the nervous over muscular nutrition, that several months were required to restore the power of locomotion. The muscles of the legs, and of the back especially, were exceedingly thin, soft and weak; it was only after these had become full and quite hard that she could walk without assistance. Her appetite, sleep, and menstruation soon became healthful. The hyperæsthesia slowly abated. All the distinctively uterine symptoms passed away with the others, without any local applications, or indeed any treatment having exclusive reference to the pelvic contents.

The issue of cases like this, when the treatment is limited to the principle of increasing nutritive action in the muscles, appears to prove the following:

That the two groups of symptoms described originate in a common cause; this cause is restricted nutrition and action of the muscles. This gives rise to both pelvic hyperæmia and to morbid nervous activity, which latter often becomes overwhelming:

That this activity takes the forms of neuralgia and hyperæsthesia:

That careful and direct mechanical stimulation of the muscles increases the amount of force for which they serve as channels:

That such stimulation increases the nutrition and size of the muscles, and thereby secures a permanent change in the relation of muscles and nerves:

That the careless, ill-advised and heterogeneous employment of the same means may prove injurious beyond remedy.

The desired results are most difficult of attainment through the agency of other remedies.

The reason is easily understood; for though there may be many drugs the effects of whose use may be to diminish the blood, and therefore the nutrition and action of the spinal cord, yet *they do not at the same time increase the nutrition and action of the muscles.* Their effects must therefore be transient, and require indefinite repetition. Obviously, what is needed in these cases is to provide some other channel besides that of the nerves through which to dispose of the force evolved by the system; and no real cure can be effected until this end is attained.

XX.

MORBID EMOTION.

The emotions furnish a channel for the exhibition of an abundance of nervous force. In the order of development the emotions are above common sensation, and appear sometimes to be but remotely connected with it. Hence emotive affections not unfrequently exist in the absence of local or persistent pain; but in its place the feelings play a very excited and often fantastic part. Popular opinion generally, and professional opinion sometimes, refer these displays of nervous action to the pelvic organs as their origin; with what propriety we will now inquire.

These nervous symptoms are included under the very objectionable and also the very indefinite term, *Hysteria.* Indefinite, because it describes nothing; objectionable, because popular opinion generally connects it with the idea of a willful perversion of intelligence, and regards its symptoms as uncontrolled rather than uncontrollable impulse. This mode of regarding hysterical symptoms may serve to quiet the otherwise anxious friends, and to reconcile the physician to the paucity of his resources; but it is inconsistent with physiology, and hinders rather than promotes a cure. As well might sciatica be supposed to be under the direct control of the will as hysteria. In radical therapeutics it is the cause of these affections whose control is sought. In hysteria there is an abundant manifestation of incoördinated force. Force is undirected or it is misdirected, and hence frequently exhibits itself in freaks. These characteristic irregularities of feeling and action simply testify to the unusual direction which the force evolved by the organism assumes. They may be as varied as the imagination can conceive. The mind may be clear, while the will is in complete abeyance; or mental action may be partly or wholly suspended. Often the intellect manifests undue excitement. The muscles may engage in violent and erratic reflex motions, or they may be quiescent. But it is the emotional powers which evidently serve as the channel for the exhibition of the force generated by the organism. The paroxysms are self-curative. The excitement is a diffusive stimulant, equalizing the circulation by transferring a portion of these energies to the muscles. This process, so far as relates to the curative intervention of muscular action, is akin to those processes or movements which may be successfully applied both as preventive and as remedial means. The relations between muscular and nervous force are thus clearly indicated. The common recourse to diffusive stimulants, and their general good though transient effects, confirm the same principle.

In this class of invalids, the connection of uterine with nervous symptoms is no more direct than in the one previously noticed. The inference is plain that their connection is through their common cause, and that medicating the pelvic contents is *not* the best method of remedying the nervous disease; for, by this course, there is a probability of exasperating the already too sensitive nerves, and thereby doing much harm.

Attacks of hysteria are referred by patient and friends to some comparatively trifling incident as cause. But the causes assigned are usually secondary, and at most provocative, rather than productive of the effect ascribed to them. The real cause is in the condition of the system, and is primarily in its habits of employing force.

In some cases there is a complete suspension of all expression of force, except such as is essential in conducting organic functions. Attacks of this kind have received the name of catalepsy. From cases that have come under my care the following is selected to illustrate and confirm the above statements : A young lady was brought to me for treatment who had for some time been subject to fits of catalepsy. She would suddenly become unconscious, and remain so for a period varying from a few minutes to two or more hours. The pulse and respiration were regular, but rather slower than usual; the countenance little changed, but wearing a vacant expression. During an attack, no reflex action could be induced by pinching or pricking any part of the body. No evidence of the activity of any of the senses could be elicited. She would lie perfectly motionless, with the exception of the heavy respiratory motion. On returning to consciousness she had no recollection of pain, or of any intellectual act. For several hours succeeding her return to the normal state she would appear weak and languid, but there was no other conspicuous evidence of ill health. She was in constant dread of these attacks, which sometimes happened daily, though generally of less frequent occurrence, and had become timid and reserved.

No medicines whatever were employed for her restoration, and no other remedy than the treatment under discussion. Abundant scope, according to her strength, was afforded her powers through the muscles. Essentially the same methods were employed as have been described already, but somewhat amplified to adapt the operations successively to the whole system, instead of confining them to those parts relating specially to the pelvis. The attacks began at once to diminish in severity, and after four weeks had ceased entirely. She has since married, has borne and lost children, but has suffered no untoward nervous symptoms.

A more recent case was that of a miss just entering upon puberty. She was a beautiful girl, free and animated in conversation, and of high intellectual development. I saw her in consultation after she had lain in bed a year almost entirely motionless. She was not raised in bed under any circumstance, for even that disturbance would excite the peculiar manifestation of her disease. Her attacks were characterized by almost perfect uniformity as to duration and manner. Each time there occurred the same motions of the facial muscles and of the arms; she uttered the same sounds, including the faint singing of snatches of two hymns; and there was the same sudden awakening to consciousness, and the same absence of sensations and memory. She usually experienced six or eight of these attacks daily, and in each of them unconsciousness lasted about two minutes.

In this instance there was activity, indicating the evolution and display of force in several disconnected channels, and its entire suppression in others. These manifestations were quite independent of intelligence, and therefore ungoverned by it. The variety and order of the displays might represent the relative facility of action of the several instruments of force.

Like other cases of this class, the disease was incurable by ordinary remedies. Medicines have more power to induce temporary suspension of vital force than to give it proper direction. At least, if there are drugs capable of affording the *permanent* control over nerve force required in such forms of disease, they are not generally known. The cure of the condition described does not require either the suspension or diminution of the force evolved by the organism, but its more correct guidance, and its application to proper uses. Such a disposition of force would effectually obviate its waste in any irregular manner.

The plan was adopted of fructifying the general muscular nutrition by means of well-directed manipulations applied by a trained assistant. The effect was gradual, but perfectly successful. I watched her progress with much interest for several weeks, during which all the symptoms diminished; and in a few months she was quite free from attacks, and had acquired very comfortable health.

The above are extreme cases of the emotive form of nervous derangement without pain. A more common class is that in which the two forms described are united in one invalid. The emotive excitement is due, in these cases, to some sudden experience of physical suffering. The one form of derangement superinduces the other. Though very obstinate or incurable, when remedial means are limited to drugs, yet experience fully justifies the statement that these cases may not only be ameliorated, but entirely cured, by carrying out the more appropriate therapeutic principles.

MORBID INTELLECTION.

The intellectual powers constitute another channel for the display of force evolved by the system. Their functions are therefore liable to be impaired by the improper distribution of force.

The particular mode of suffering to which attention is now called is mental subordination. Intellectual acts cease to be of first importance—morbid sensation and emotion assume a place above them. The feelings bear undisputed sway in the formation of judgment. Thought is hence persistently guided in a wrong direction, and becomes centred on interior bodily organs. It is controlled by subjective impressions. It is so much directed within that it has little effective objective power.

This condition is shown in various and often contradictory ways. The invalid becomes a martyr to petty and inconsequent notions—perhaps regarding her personal comforts, or her relations with others. She is assertive and inflexible, especially with reference to the limitation of her powers, her conclusions being strictly controlled by her *feelings*. Her ideas and statements concerning herself are the combined product of paramount sensation and emotion and the subordinated intellectual powers; and while they are the exact reflex of the predominating nervous activity, they are quite unreliable as to her actual physical state. Extreme pain in a region of the body, or suspension of its use, indicates the modes in which the sensations report to the intelligence, rather than its actual condition.

An instance of these aberrations of mental and sensorial power was that of a well-educated young lady, of good physical appearance, who could walk about the city without discomfort, and make daily excursions to neighboring places of resort; yet she imagined that she could neither actually sit nor lie. Her favorite and almost exclusive position was reclining upon one elbow, the head supported by the hand. She was distressed when she changed from this position, and nothing could prevail upon her long to deviate from it. She had been for three or four years treated locally for uterine affections, and complained of many symptoms referable to the pelvis, but a thorough examination revealed no physical evidence of disease in that region. It was evident that the pelvis, the sensations, emotions and intellect all suffered from the same cause; and that this cause was the undue and prolonged preponderance of nerve over muscular activity, and from the reflection of this force interiorly, instead of its normal expenditure upon exterior objects.

It is probable that in this case the condition described was promoted, if not caused, by repeated local applications. There can be no doubt that the ultimate effect of many such applications is to superinduce sensitiveness of the pelvic nerves, and of the spinal centres connected therewith. This is sufficient to make the pelvis a point of convergence of mental action. Prolonged pain fixes the attention upon the suffering region. The mind thus readily acquires a habit of receiving and responding to subjective impressions, but has no data whereby to estimate their value. Hence insignificant causes often produce effects as grave as those more formidable.

These and many other peculiarities in the manifestation of nerve force, when properly interpreted, do not denote conscious, much less willful, perversity. Neither do they indicate a serious degree of organic imperfection. They are evidences of functional excesses and deficiencies. They imply a pre-engagement of the limited power which the system generates; a restriction to and excess in a narrow channel, leaving that which should be traversed quite unoccupied, or the inward instead of an outward direction to the forces generated by the system.

This is the reverse of the natural and healthful disposition of bodily power. The organism is adapted to expend its forces exteriorly as a condition of their continuance. It yields its power as a luminous body does its effulgence. If the direction be reversed, and the force designed for exterior uses be applied to interior processes, it becomes a powerful agency for disturbing organic nutritive operations. The consequences of this improper direction of nervous power are shown in the restricted amount and deteriorated quality of the manifestation afforded. Preoccupied with sensations having a subjective origin, the mind can command but little power for other uses.

The reason invalids of the class here described soon become and continue helpless, is now apparent. In proportion to the mental introversion is their inaptitude for exertion. The brain, organs of sense and feeling, overact; therefore the muscles must act feebly, if at all. This condition becomes habitual and second nature. Indeed, any intimation of the necessity for muscular action is often regarded by these invalids as a decided indication of unfriendliness. Their judgment is almost entirely subordinated to their feelings.

The degree of this preponderance of nerve over muscular power and action is sometimes such that the invalid scarcely exists as an object representing dynamic power, but endures a manifold existence, in combined sensation, emotion and excited mental action. The purposes of physical existence are to a degree subverted; for dynamic power—that which overcomes physical obstacles—is the first necessity of existence, and the leading function of all animated beings. Indeed, all physical beings except those of the human species soon pass out of existence when deprived of it. The superior endurance of the human race is shown in the fact that the human female will continue to exist for an indefinite period after being almost wholly deprived of physical power.

To persons accustomed to consider disease solely in its relations with material remedies, these views may appear fanciful. But experience has fairly proved that such remedies fall short of their aim, when this aim is the control of nervous function.

Disease evidently relates to the uses of the body, as well as to its materials. It cannot legitimately be restricted to effects and products. Function and purpose are not material. A hand is raised; by this act the superiority and the control of vital force is asserted not only over gravitation, which impels the limb in an opposite direction, but also over the elements which constitute the series of organic cells by which the power thus manifested has been evolved. This vital force is the agency whose misapplication or partial suppression is the primary and essential element in the form of disease under consideration. It is an element of disease, because it is also an element of health. Its importance in the one case can no more be questioned than in the other. That it can be employed to restore health is no more improbable than that it can be used to maintain health.

The difference in the manifestation and use of corporeal force in health and in disease is, that in the former case there is a perfect counterpoise of the different forms of its expression; in the latter, there is not. The exercise of the various bodily powers serve as mutual checks upon each other, preventing excess. No form of power can reach its proper expression if not duly related to other forms. Or, to reduce the idea to its practical statement, health of the nervous system can neither be restored nor maintained without the counterpoise of muscular action.

The truth now stated is essentially impregnable, scarcely admitting of exceptions; but its full confirmation by experience requires much time. This is because disease accrues gradually, though the symptoms may develop rapidly. Indeed, diseases of the kind now discussed almost always date much farther back than the patient and friends are willing to acknowledge. Prolonged disease acquires an additional power, that of habit, which adds greatly to the difficulty of overcoming it. The disease becomes incorporated in the very structures, is daily reproduced in the nutritive processes, and becomes, in fact, constitutional. Only by reversing the processes by which disease is acquired, can it be removed.

RESTORATION OF HELPLESS INVALIDS.

To restore those who have been long prostrated on beds of suffering with diseases to which this work is specially devoted, is a matter of no secondary importance. And it is no wonder if the judgment of friends is somewhat staggered by the various and conflicting methods that the medical art proposes to secure this end. In my method the restoration of power seems to the invalid to be spontaneous; there is no tasking of inadequate powers, no crisis to pass, no unnatural and inordinate effort to be made. Health comes from the supply to the invalid of two chief deficiencies of which she has long been abundantly conscious. First, the capacity for *evolving* force; second, the capacity for *directing* force. As soon as these *capacities* are developed, the work is essentially accomplished.

It is simply futile for the physician to attempt the direction, or the invalid to attempt the use, of power which does not exist. But as soon as a helpless invalid *feels* the thrill of increased warmth in, and flow of blood and nervous power to the extremities, then she feels a consciousness of increased capacity, and *desires* to use it. She does not hang back, does not wait for moral incentives, requires no extraordinary stimulus to employ her powers or to awaken her consciousness of their possession. Those who have employed the aid of crutches or the physical assistance of others are too happy in foregoing their use, and rejoice in their emancipation. No artificial supports, no braces of any kind, are needed, even in the first essays of strength. An invalid delights in the use of her newly-developed powers as surely as the child delights in its triumph of standing and walking. Rational incentives become as supererogatory in the one case as the other.

ORIGIN AND PREDISPOSING CAUSES OF NERVOUS DERANGEMENT IN FEMALES.

Children inherit feeble muscles, and display from the commencement of life predominant nervous activity. This is a perfectly natural consequence of the use to which the parents apply *their* powers. No law is more incontrovertible than that "like begets like." This transmission is not confined to constitution, but extends to *habit*—the occupations of the different channels of force.

It follows that habitual strain of the nervous system of parents will be liable to superinduce an unnatural tension of nerves in offspring; and this will be wholly irrespective of original soundness of constitution in the parents.

This being admitted, the necessity of early endeavors to counteract this inborn tendency to excessive nervous activity and irritability in children is apparent. But parents are unwilling practically to admit the deteriorating influence of their own nervous habits on their children. They prefer to place an undue estimate on the presumedly favorable, constitutional, hereditary traits. They do not understand the importance of such repression on the one side, and cultivation on the other, as shall insure an equipoise in the manifestation of force by their children. They are foolishly vain of the precocity of their children, and take little or no pains to repress this sure evidence of the morbid preponderance of nervous action. On the contrary, they are inclined to stimulate all indications of precocity, and thus increase the activity of the already too excited nerves. The consequence is, that vital force is in this way prodigally expended, when it should be reserved for normal use and muscular growth.

Such reserve of power is quite capable of being attained for even weakly children through intelligent cultivation, and the importance to parents of understanding the proper means for this cannot be overestimated. The consequences of neglect are disastrous. Reserve power does not congenitally exist, and as none has been acquired by due training for that special purpose, it follows that such children have deficient physical stamina, and cannot combat with success the diseases of childhood, to which large numbers prove early victims.

In childhood, the girl begins to fall behind the boy in point of physical advantages. While the boy is allowed to royster about the streets and fields, expanding his chest, hardening his muscles, increasing his physical capacity, and acquiring reserve of force against future emergencies, the girl is practically excluded from equal, or even any adequate, advantage for physical development. Instead of being encouraged to engage in invigorating exercises, she is taught propriety of demeanor, which, unfortunately for her, generally is of a sort which not only represses all outflow of force through the muscles, but includes abundant stimulus for the emotions and other forms of nervous activity.

Education now steps in, and with refined and often cruel skill gives a further preponderance to the intellectual and sensorial faculties. Physical culture, instead of being pushed forward in commensurate degree, is utterly neglected. Young women know nothing of its methods, purposes, possibilities, or ends. The little that is incidentally presented to them in the form of household occupations they have learned to avoid and contemn. They are not, by the dictum of society, allowed even the poor advantage of self-helpfulness. The grossest ignorance of the most uncultivated people affords the physical powers of women better advantages than is practically bestowed by our enlightenment.

At the age of puberty comes a serious test of the consequences of allowing the want of equipoise of nervous and muscular activity to exist.

This is a period when nature makes an attempt to manifest an exuberance of animal life. The degree of success with which this is achieved attests the nature and degree of the preparation. In case of preponderant nervous development this attempt is a partial failure, and various untoward symptoms occur, the first fruits of the seed early sown. Muscular weakness and nervous excitement are no longer the only difficulties. These, in fact, are now lost sight of and their existence is forgotten, in the presence of their more serious consequences. It is the weak if not the deformed spine, the delicate lungs, the inactive stomach, the neuralgia, the hysteria or some of the forms of uterine disease that engross the attention of friends and physicians, instead of defective dynamic energy and misapplied nutrition. But these primary causes nevertheless exist in unabated degree. The secondary series of affections will necessarily continue, while the primary, upon which they wholly depend, shall remain. The value of the remainder of life is now seriously impaired. From this time forward these unfortunate individuals are the fluctuating subjects of hope and despair, attributing their suffering to some mysterious trouble with their pelvic organs.

Closely connected with this period in the order of nature is the development of the emotional powers; those powers which, manifested as affections, are capable of subduing man and the world. At no time does the female more need a goodly fund of reserve power; and even when thus endowed, there are those who require the cautious direction of experienced heads and hearts to maintain equipoise, and thus prevent the wreck of the nervous system. Instead of this, however, her associations impel her in one direction. There is provided for her reading, called light, but which arouses the emotions and sharpens the senses; society with its ambitions, its rivalries and its blandishments; music and the refined arts;—all of which are good and desirable in their way and place and at proper times, but none of them provide for the stern realities about to dawn upon her. What is most needed in her case is an ample resource of physical power for the immediate future. Without such provision, life's struggles and pains will be abundantly suffered, increased and intensified, while its successes and joys will be reserved solely for stronger constitutions. The chief aim of life, *money*, is found on trial to be no compensation for the chief need of life, *power;* the muscles have not been trained for life's occasions.

It is not therefore strange or unnatural that when marriage comes there is no adequate preparation for its duties, much less for its emergencies. The young woman may be emotionally, sensorially and intellectually cultivated; but the higher the degree of these forms of life, the more unfitted she is apt to be for the position she is now to assume as wife and mother. These are not all the important qualifications she and her family need to find in her. She tries to perform her new duties by the aid of her only available faculties, those of thought and emotion. But these are not available in the direction desired, and only more intense and painful thinking and feeling are the results of her efforts.

The forces evolved in her endeavor cannot travel through muscles, for these channels have scarcely more than a supposable existence. In proportion to this muscular deficiency is this excess of perverted nervous activity, and the development of the disease which has long existed potentially in her system.

If weakness of muscle, excited but unproductive nervous action, and pelvic disorder were the deliberately intended result of the rearing of women, this result could hardly be more surely and fully attained than it is by the usual course pursued in the education of girls. The ill health which so regularly occurs is not spontaneous, nor the result of fortuitious circumstances. No other consequence could well follow the causes. As disease is the product of prolonged defective training, so may recovery also be the product of correct training. What more reasonable than the proposition that opposite causes will produce opposite effects?

GLOSSARY.

Abnormal. Unhealthy, unnatural.
Adipose. Fatty.
Alterative. Medicines which re-establish the healthy functions of the system.
Amenorrhœa. Suppression or retention of menses.
Anœmia. An impoverished state of the blood.
Anæsthesia. Diminution of sense of feeling.
Anteversion. Bending forward.
Antiphlogistic. Remedy against inflammation.
Aperient. Medicine which gently opens the bowels.
Areolar. Containing *areolæ*—small spaces between fibres composing organs.
Capillaries. Hair-like vessels for conveying the blood from the arteries to the veins.
Catalepsy. Sudden suppression of will and senses,—trunk and limbs taking and retaining any fixed position.
Cellular. Composed of cells.
Cellulitis. Inflammation of cellular tissues.
Cervical. Pertaining to the neck.
Coccyx. Bones forming lower end of spinal column.
Concomitant. A companion; a person or thing that accompanies another.
Congestion. Over-fullness of blood-vessels.
Co-ordination. Equal standing in the same relation to something higher or lower.
Diagnosis. Determining the disease.
Diaphragm. The large breathing muscle between chest and abdomen.
Dynamic. Pertaining to strength and power.
Dyscrasy. An evil habit of body.
Edematous. Swelling.
Endometrial. Within the womb.
Enema. Injection into the rectum.
Epigastric. Belonging to the epigastrium, that part of the abdomen immediately over the stomach.
Etiology. The science of the cause of disease.
Function. The office or duty of an organ.
Gynecology. The science which treats of the female constitution.

Hygiene. The art of preserving health.
Hyperæmia. More than a natural amount of blood in the capillaries.
Hyperæsthesia. Excessive sensibility.
Hypersecretion. Excessive secretion.
Hypertrophy. Excessive growth or thickening of an organ.
Idiopathic. Relating to *idiopathy*—a disease arising spontaneously.
Interstitial. Situated between; pertaining to interstices.
Introversion. Turned within.
Lumbar. Pertaining to the loins.
Menorrhagia. Excessive menstruation.
Mesenteric. The membrane which retains the intestines and appendages in position.
Metrial. Pertaining to the womb.
Metamorphosis. Transformation.
Metritis. Inflammation of the womb.
Nidus. Nest.
Os. Mouth.
Osmotic. Pertaining to osmose; the action by which fluids pass through a porous solid.
Parenchyma. The texture of glandular organs, as the liver, etc.
Pathological. Morbid changes.
Pathology. That which explains the nature and cause of disease.
Physiology. The science of living beings.
Potentially. In possibility; not positively.
Prolification. Act of bearing offspring.
Proximate. Nearest.
Reciprocatory. Interchanging
Retroverted. Bent backward.
Retroactive. Acting back.
Sacral. Pertaining to the sacrum, the large triangular bone at the end of the spinal column.
Sanguineous. Bloody.
Sensory. Connected with sensation.
Strumous. Scrofulous.
Therapeutics. The treatment of disease.
Tissue. The peculiar structure of a part.
Topical. Local.
Toxic. Poisonous.
Uterus. The womb.
Vagina. The passage leading to the womb.
Viscera. The entrails.

www.ingramcontent.com/pod-product-compliance
Lightning Source LLC
LaVergne TN
LVHW020224110826
845151LV00003B/819

* 9 7 8 1 4 2 5 5 3 2 2 6 0 *